Sex in The Villages

Sex in The Villages

Unconventional Tips to Enhance Sexual Health and Wellness in Retirement

Tina M. Penhollow, Ph.D.

Contents

Introduction

Welcome to *Sex in The Villages*—your guide to living a vibrant and passionate life as you age! Get ready to transform your view of life after 55. This book goes beyond offering advice; it's a practical guide packed with science-based strategies to enhance every aspect of your daily living. If you want to increase your energy, find more joy, and enjoy a satisfying sex life, this book is for you.

Life in The Villages is anything but ordinary. Picture the gentle hum of golf carts, the calm of poolside relaxation, and the lively energy of countless social events. This palm-lined paradise is a vibrant, self-contained haven where retirees focus on making the most of every moment.

After over 20 years of exploring this unique community, I've gathered many insights through personal experiences and extensive research. In these pages, you'll meet fascinating individuals and hear their stories while discovering practical tips to help you enjoy and thrive in this exciting chapter of life.

Whether you're a proud resident of The Villages or simply seeking ways to enhance your well-being, this book equips you with the tools to elevate your sexual health and overall vitality.

Let's challenge the outdated myths about sexuality in later life and embrace the rewarding experiences that come with aging. The Villages is more than just a destination; it's a way of living where growing older is an exciting journey to be celebrated.

Join me as we uncover the secrets to living a life filled with passion, joy, and endless possibilities!

CHAPTER 1

The "Boomer Bubble"

"Sex in retirement isn't about recapturing youth; it's about embracing the fullness of life at every stage."

— Jane Fonda, American Actress

Living in a Bubble

The Villages is the largest active retirement community in the world—a popular destination for people aged 55 and older. Located in central Florida, this vibrant community is often called "Adult Disneyland" because of its lively and fun-loving residents. With an average age of 66, it's the perfect place for those who feel young at heart. Beneath its peaceful exterior lies a world of endless excitement and surprises.

Primarily home to affluent white retirees, The Villages combines Florida's unique charm with a lively atmosphere, making it a one-of-a-kind retirement experience. It has gained attention for its golf cart rendezvous, adventurous lifestyle, and higher-than-average rates of sexually transmitted infections (STIs)—even the New York Post has given it the playful tagline "ground zero for geriatrics who are seriously getting it on."

History and Overview

The community's story began in the 1970s when Harold Schwartz and Al Tarrson purchased a large plot of land in the middle of Florida. What started as a peaceful retirement spot soon became a magnet for those seeking a lively and social retirement. Today, The Villages has grown to house over 145,000 residents, making it the fastest-growing metro area in the U.S. over the last decade.

Within The Villages, you'll find a self-sufficient community designed to keep you engaged and worry-free. Residents start their day with The Daily Sun, the community's newspaper, which delivers only positive news (because who needs negativity in paradise?). Local TV stations provide entertainment and information to keep everyone in the loop.

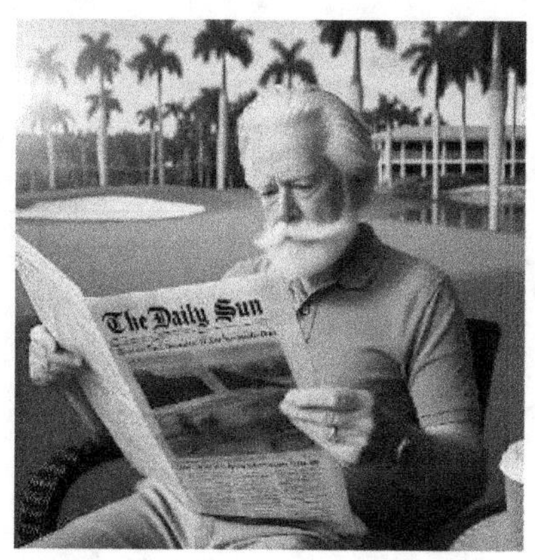

Your safety is paramount, with police and fire stations always ready to help—without intrusive sirens to disturb your peace. Your health and wellness are top priorities, with hospitals, pharmacies, wellness centers, and schools conveniently located within the community. No cemeteries are located within The Villages—after all, this place is for the living! Every detail is designed to create a seamless, joyful living experience just for you.

A resident once said, "Once you arrive in The Villages, age is just a number—we're all the same." This statement reflects the community's environment, where age truly doesn't matter. Neighbors form close bonds, living by the phrase, "Birds of a feather flock together." This tight-knit community fosters a warm and inviting atmosphere. Still, it can also create a sense of isolation from the outside world. Life inside The Villages is so fulfilling that residents often feel little need to venture out.

This community is a playground for Baby Boomers, a generation celebrated for its zest for life and adventurous spirit. Having lived through transformative decades, they've experienced it all—and perhaps indulged in more than a few unforgettable escapades along the way! In The Villages, they've cleverly created their lively world, fondly known as "The Boomer

Bubble." Here, they celebrate their shared past, make new memories, and enjoy a spirited lifestyle that only this unique group can create.

Discussions about sex and aging have become more common in The Villages. What was once a taboo topic is now considered necessary for overall health. Engaging in open and honest discussions cultivates a welcoming and supportive environment that empowers residents to feel more confident and comfortable as they navigate the unique challenges of aging and sexual well-being.

As you dive deeper into the topic of sexuality in The Villages, it's essential to recognize that sexual health is a critical component of overall well-being at any age. With dating sites and social clubs for single older adults, this community has become a place where people explore new relationships and embrace their sexuality later in life.

Living the Dream

The Villages offers countless amenities designed for fun, relaxation, and fulfillment. Spanning 51,200 acres, this retirement haven boasts 35 community centers and over 3,000 clubs, ensuring there's always something exciting to do. With a vibrant social scene, diverse recreational activities, and top-notch amenities—this community truly stands out as unique.

State-of-the-art fitness centers with the latest exercise machines, group fitness classes, and personal training options can be found throughout the community. You'll also find over 100 indoor and outdoor swimming pools—perfect for relaxation, water aerobics, and lap swimming. The extensive network of walking and biking trails also invites you to stay active while soaking in the sun amid the beautiful tropical scenery.

If you love golf, The Villages is a dream come true! With 56 golf courses and 711 holes, this community offers more golfing opportunities than any other community or facility in the world. Golf carts, often called "golf cars" by the locals, are the primary mode of transportation. With around 60,000 of these vehicles zipping through town, they are essential to daily life. These carts provide a convenient and charming way to navigate the community's vast paths and streets. More Yamaha golf carts are sold here than anywhere else in the U.S.

Pickleball is another popular sport in The Villages, which has earned the unofficial title of "Pickleball Capital of the World." With over 300 dedicated pickleball courts and more regularly added, there are plenty of chances to improve your game and join in friendly yet competitive matches. The lively pickleball community provides many opportunities for social interaction, physical fitness, and fun.

Healthcare in The Villages

Healthcare in The Villages is designed to meet all your needs and ensure you have access to high-quality medical care. The community offers a variety of facilities, including primary care centers, specialized clinics, and hospitals—all of which aim to provide convenient and excellent services.

A key provider in the area is The Villages Health. This network of primary care centers is spread throughout the community, making it easy to see

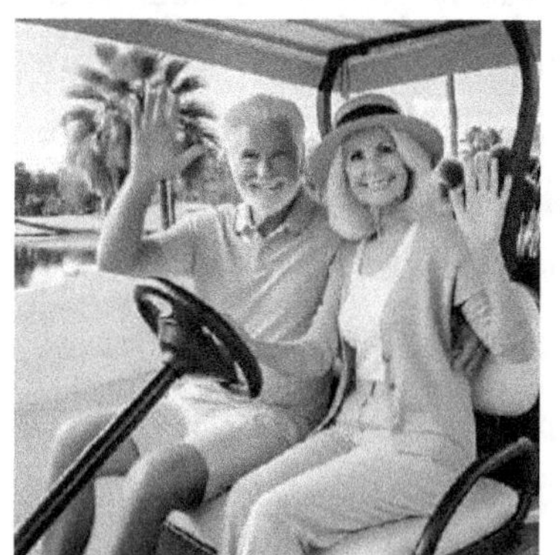

general practitioners and family medicine doctors. These centers focus on preventive care, managing chronic diseases, and offering wellness programs with a patient-centered approach.

Primary care centers are your go-to for routine check-ups, vaccinations, and managing ongoing health conditions. They help you stay on top of your health with regular screenings and personalized care plans. Specialized clinics offer expert cardiology, orthopedics, and dermatology care for more specific needs, ensuring you receive specialized attention when necessary.

Hospitals in The Villages are equipped with state-of-the-art technology and staffed by highly trained professionals, ensuring they are well-prepared to address serious health issues and emergencies. Offering a wide range of comprehensive services, from emergency care to advanced surgeries, these hospitals provide high-quality treatment, allowing you to receive the care you need without traveling far from home.

Preventive care is a primary focus in The Villages, with numerous programs designed to keep you healthy and active. Wellness programs offer fitness classes, nutrition advice, and health education. Chronic disease management programs provide ongoing support and treatment for conditions like diabetes, high blood pressure, and heart disease. So, whether you need a routine check-up, specialized care, or emergency treatment—you can be confident in receiving excellent and convenient care.

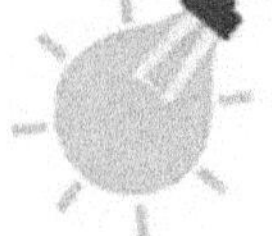

Clubs, Groups, and Games

The social scene is vibrant and energetic in The Villages! With over 3,000 special interest clubs covering hobbies like gardening, photography, and travel, you'll have plenty of opportunities to meet new people and build connections that enhance your social well-being. Joining groups focused on interests such as painting, glassmaking, and woodworking allows you to connect with others who share your passions. Participating in community activities helps you make friends, reduce feelings of loneliness, and improve your mental well-being.

A long-term study of older adults in the U.S. found that those who stayed socially active lived much longer over the 13 years of the study compared to those who were less active. This highlights the importance of social engagement in later life, showing that factors beyond physical fitness contribute to better overall health status. Adults in the study who stayed socially, mentally, and physically active were those who aged most successfully.

Staying mentally active and socially engaged is easy with the many games and hobbies available. Game rooms offer spaces for card games, board games, and billiards. At the same time, hobby clubs cater to interests like model building, bird watching, and stamp collecting. Book clubs and discussion groups meet regularly to talk about literature, current events, philosophy, and history, offering intellectual stimulation and social interaction.

Exploring your creative side through arts and crafts can be very rewarding. Art studios offer facilities for painting, sculpture, and ceramics, allowing you to express yourself artistically. Craft workshops provide classes in woodworking, jewelry making, sewing, and other skills, where you can learn new techniques and meet like-minded individuals.

Regular social gatherings and themed parties, such as holiday celebrations and costume parties, create festive atmospheres that encourage deeper relationships. Mixers and dances, including ballroom and line dancing, allow singles and couples to connect and socialize.

Travel and excursions let you explore new places and experiences, helping you build friendships and maybe even romance. You can join organized day trips to local attractions, parks, and cultural sites or join travel clubs for group trips across the U.S. and worldwide. These activities broaden your horizons and help you form lasting relationships.

Dr. Penhollow (yes, that's me!) and colleagues conducted a study in The Villages, uncovering some interesting findings about social activities. Among the women, 19% said they participate in social activities daily, and 65% reported joining in at least once a week. Only 16% said they don't participate in any social events. For men, 12% were involved in daily social activities, 64% joined at least weekly, and 24% reported taking part less often. These numbers show that while many residents are very active in community life, others prefer a more laid-back, less frequent approach to socializing.

Tips:

- **Explore The Villages:** Dive into the vibrant community of The Villages, where rich history and a lively social scene come together. Connect with long-time residents to hear their personal stories and gain valuable tips on maintaining a healthy and fulfilling sexual life. Their experiences might inspire you and add a new spark to your relationships and overall well-being.

- **Stay Active and Engaged:** Keep your life dynamic by joining clubs and social groups. These activities help you stay physically fit and socially connected. By staying engaged with your community and participating in activities that keep you moving, you'll find that your overall well-being—including your sexual health—thrives.

CHAPTER 2

The "Loofah Code"

"The only unnatural sex act is that which you cannot perform."
— Alfred Kinsey, American Sexologist

Inside The Villages' Culture

The Villages, often called "America's Friendliest Hometown," is celebrated for its energetic and dynamic community. Known for its lively social scene, it stands out for promoting a vibrant and engaging atmosphere that encourages connection and active living.

Headlines about public sex incidents and related arrests have contributed to the community's somewhat notorious reputation for a lively and occasionally controversial social scene. The Villages made headlines when two residents were arrested for engaging in public sex at Lake Sumter Landing, a well-known town square, witnessed by several people, including families. Other incidents have involved couples in compromising situations on golf courses, public parks, and parking lots. This has drawn significant media attention and sparked discussions about the community's social norms. There have also been reports of arrests for solicitation, where individuals were accused of offering or engaging in sexual services for money.

There's also a more private side to its social scene, including swingers and "loofahs." Yes, you read that right—golf clubs aren't the only things swinging in this community!

In 2008, The Villages ran an advertising campaign that unexpectedly added to its colorful reputation. The direct mail promotion aimed to attract new residents by sending promotional materials, including a free loofah sponge. While the gift was intended to be practical, the loofah sparked some surprising reactions.

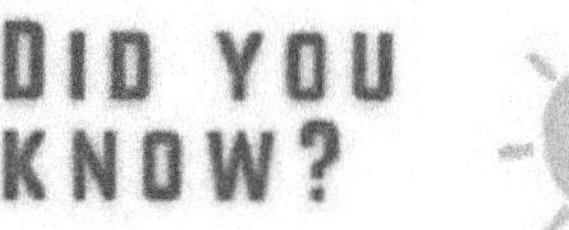
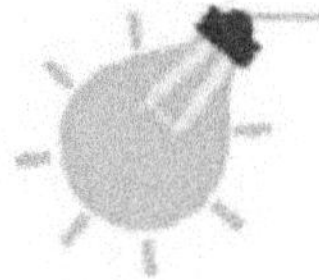

Online communities and social groups dedicated to swinging lifestyles are increasingly popular among older adults

Some recipients interpreted the loofah as suggestive and inappropriate, associating it with personal hygiene and bathing—speculating that it hinted at sexual activities. Critics argued that the campaign misrepresented the lifestyle of The Villages' residents, especially among older adults.

The controversy around the loofahs led to discussions about the community's culture and whether using potential sexual innuendos in marketing materials was appropriate for an older audience. Although the administration did not intend for the loofahs to be seen in a sexual context, the incident sparked debates about the community's image and marketing strategies.

While The Villages has distanced itself from the loofah controversy, this quirky chapter remains a notable part of its history. It's often referenced in discussions about the community's lively social scene and active residents.

Should you venture into this vibrant community, it's important to recognize and appreciate its lively, often provocative essence. The very elements that stir debate are also what makes it so uniquely captivating and intriguing.

Rumors, Scandals, and Swinging

Persistent rumors suggest that some village residents participate in swinging activities. Swingers are people or couples who engage in consensual, non-monogamous relationships, often exchanging partners with others who share the same interests. While these activities are typically private, they can become a topic of conversation and speculation in close-knit communities like The Villages.

The "Loofah Code"

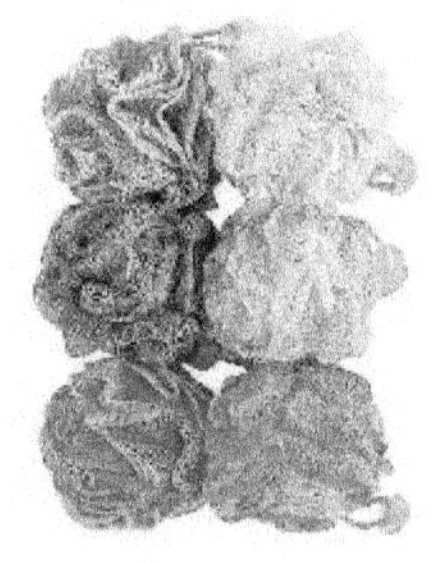

In The Villages, the "loofah code" is a term used to describe a supposed communication system among swingers. Instead of using the traditional upside-down pineapple, residents are said to use loofahs (or similar items like colored ribbons, pool noodles, or pom-poms) attached to their golf carts to signal their interest in swinging. Different colors reportedly represent various preferences or availability for activities.

Here's a fun breakdown of the loofah code:

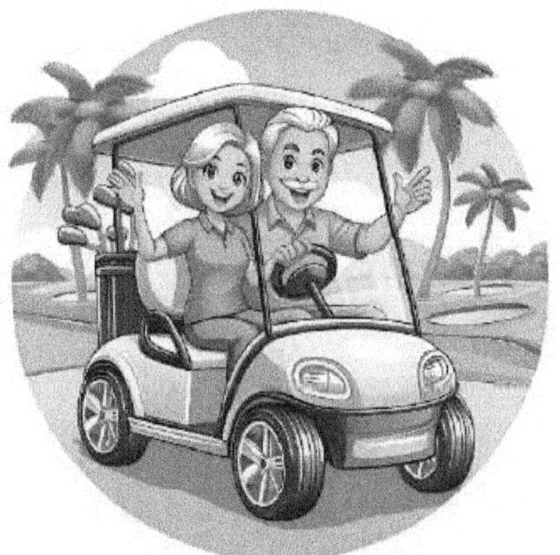

- **White:** Novice (beginner)

- **Purple:** Voyeur (people who like to watch)

- **Pink:** Soft swap (kissing)

- **Blue:** Full swap and same-room swap (penetration but in the same room)

- **Yellow:** Mid-level swap (full swap with more involved activities, but perhaps still in the same room)

- **Black:** Full swap (different room, partner exchange)

- **Teal:** Bisexual (for those who want to increase their dating chances)

A study by the North American Swing Club Association (NASCA) surveyed 1,000 married, white, upper-middle-class, middle-aged, church-going individuals and found that 15% of couples in the U.S. have tried swinging at some point. It's estimated that 2-4% of married couples swing occasionally. Interestingly, many participants reported that swinging increased their marital happiness, with swinging couples rating their marriage and overall life satisfaction higher than those who don't swing.

Decoding Community Dynamics

As a resident or visitor, you might find the rumors and practices in The Villages intriguing. Swinging, which often sparks curiosity and conversation, is a deeply personal choice for those who participate. In a close-knit community like The Villages, discretion and respect for others' choices are crucial. Whether or not these activities appeal to you, they illustrate the diverse ways people seek connection and happiness in their relationships.

The rumors about swinging and the so-called "loofah code" highlight the complex social dynamics of The Villages. While local gossip and media outlets have popularized the idea of a loofah code, much of this is based on hearsay and needs more solid evidence. Many residents may simply use loofahs to locate their golf carts. The loofah code might be more of an urban legend or playful myth than a widespread practice—although that's up to you to decide!

As a large retirement community with a diverse population, The Villages offers a range of social activities and lifestyles. While some residents may engage in unconventional sexual activities, others may prefer a more traditional approach. Stories about swingers and the loofah code add an intriguing layer to the community's reputation. Nevertheless, The Villages remains a popular and vibrant destination for retirees, providing numerous activities and social opportunities.

Now, here's the intriguing information you've been waiting for! According to the data, about 3% of residents in The Villages identify

These numbers reveal that some residents in The Villages are open to exploring different relationship styles, showcasing the community's acceptance and diversity. This willingness to try non-traditional relationships highlights how inclusive and vibrant life in The Villages can be. The Villages isn't just about traditional social interactions—it's also a place where individuals feel comfortable exploring and expressing their unique preferences. This variety enriches the community, creating an environment where different lifestyles can thrive together.

Tips:

- **Avoid Rumors:** In a close-knit community like The Villages, it's easy for rumors to spread. Don't let gossip cloud your judgment or affect your relationships. Focus on getting to know people directly and form your own opinions. Keeping a positive mindset and steering clear of rumors will help you build stronger, more meaningful connections with those around you.

- **Respect Alternative Lifestyles:** The Villages is home to diverse individuals with different backgrounds and lifestyles, including various sexual orientations and preferences. Embrace this diversity by respecting others' choices and being open-minded. Acknowledging and accepting alternative sexual lifestyles contributes to a more inclusive, supportive, and harmonious community where everyone can feel valued and respected.

CHAPTER 3

Sexology 101

"The only way to deal with fear is to face it head-on. The only way to understand sex is to learn about it openly."

— Sigmund Freud, Founder of Psychoanalysis

The Many Facets of Sexual Health

Sexual health involves much more than just the physical—it's a blend of emotional, mental, social, and cultural well-being that evolves over time. By nurturing each of these areas, you can navigate the changes that come with age and keep your intimate relationships fulfilling and vibrant. Embracing these aspects allows you to better understand your own needs and continue enjoying a deeply connected, satisfying life. In this chapter, let's take a closer look at the essential dimensions of sexual health and discover how they work together to support your journey to a confident, joyful sense of intimacy.

Physical Health

Your physical health forms the foundation of a satisfying and balanced sexual life. Staying active and prioritizing your fitness can boost your stamina, flexibility, and energy, all of which can positively influence your intimate life. Engaging in regular exercise, eating well, and managing any health conditions help you feel strong and capable, adding to a more fulfilling and enjoyable intimate experience. Physical health isn't just about looks—it's about feeling comfortable and confident in your body, which can elevate your self-esteem and enhance your sexual enjoyment.

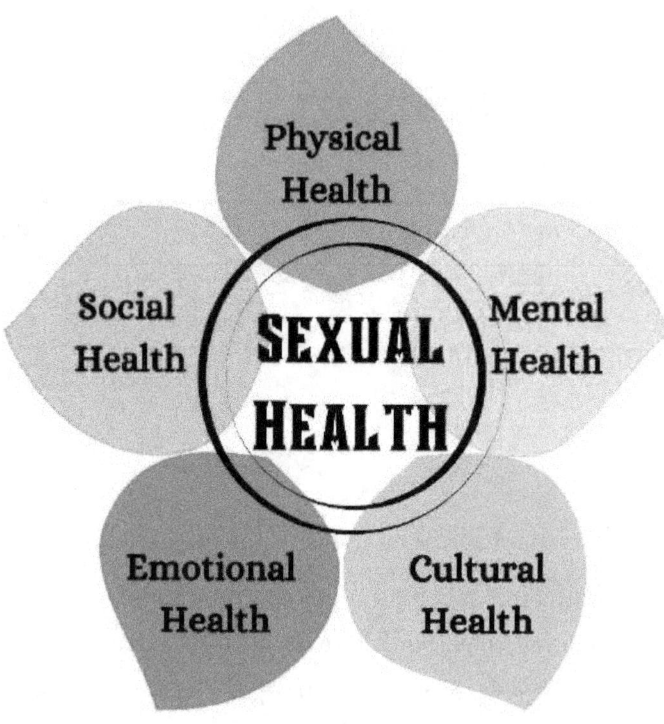

Emotional Health

Your emotional well-being plays a vital role in your sexual health, especially as you grow older. The way you feel emotionally influences the quality of your intimate relationships. Nurturing close connections—whether with friends, family, or a partner—can deepen your sense of intimacy and togetherness. Recognizing and understanding your emotions, from joy to frustration, helps you communicate openly and feel more satisfied in your relationships. Prioritizing your emotional health not only lifts your mood and outlook but also enhances your intimate experiences, allowing you to feel more connected, confident, and fulfilled.

Mental Health

Your mental well-being is essential to a fulfilling sexual life, particularly as you adapt to the changes that come with aging. How you view yourself and your relationships shapes your overall sexual health. Cultivating a positive outlook, managing stress effectively, and keeping your mind engaged all contribute to a richer, more satisfying intimate life. By nurturing your mental health, you're better equipped to face challenges, communicate clearly, and embrace confidence in expressing yourself. Prioritizing mental wellness helps ease any anxiety or self-doubt—allowing you to connect deeply with others, enjoy meaningful intimacy, and find greater satisfaction in your relationships.

Social Health

Social health is a vital aspect of your sexual health, particularly as you grow older. Building and sustaining positive connections with friends, family, and your community fosters a sense of belonging and emotional stability. Staying socially active allows you to share experiences, deepen connections, and build trust—all of which lead to more rewarding relationships. When you invest in your social health, you feel more supported, confident, and open to expressing your needs and desires. Engaging with others brings companionship, joy, and stronger emotional bonds, all of which enhance your overall sense of intimacy and satisfaction.

Cultural Health

Cultural health is a vital yet often underappreciated part of sexual health. The values, beliefs, and traditions you carry shape how you view intimacy and relationships. Embracing your cultural identity and respecting diverse viewpoints can significantly enrich your sexual health. Cultural awareness fosters open-mindedness, giving you insight into how your background and life experiences influence your approach to intimacy. By connecting with your heritage, you cultivate confidence in expressing yourself in relationships. When you honor your roots and engage with people from different cultures, you broaden your understanding of sexual health, enhancing the depth and fulfillment of your intimate life.

Myths, Taboos, and Truths

Even though we live in an era of unprecedented openness, society often lags when it comes to attitudes about sexuality later in life. Ageist stereotypes and taboos often cast a shadow over discussions about sexuality—spreading myths and misconceptions that can have real, adverse effects. Even in progressive retirement communities like The Villages, stereotypes often prevail, making it difficult to have open and honest conversations. It's crucial to address these biases to ensure you enjoy a fulfilling and healthy sex life free from outdated and harmful assumptions.

Myth 1: Sex Isn't Important for Older Adults

A common misconception is that sexual desire naturally diminishes with age, as though interest in intimacy has an expiration date. This myth fails to recognize the wide spectrum of sexual experiences and desires that can flourish throughout one's life. In truth, many people maintain vibrant and fulfilling sex lives well into their later years. Unfortunately, this stereotype can lead to the false assumption that older adults don't need or want sexual health support and care. Breaking down this myth is crucial to ensuring you receive the comprehensive sexual health attention you deserve.

Myth 2: Older Adults Lose Interest in Sex

Another widespread myth suggests that sex is only for the young and only youthful bodies and daring spirits can truly enjoy it. This belief dismisses the reality that sexuality is a lifelong journey, one that evolves and deepens with age. Many older adults remain curious about their sexuality and are eager to try new experiences—whether through experimenting with different techniques, exploring intimacy aids, or simply finding new ways to connect. Your sexual needs and desires deserve respect and support without judgment or age-based stereotypes. Recognizing the diversity of experiences among older adults highlights the importance of sexual expression at every stage of life. No matter your age, intimacy and connection are essential to your happiness and well-being.

Myth 3: Older Adults Are Not at Risk for STIs

A common misconception is that sexually transmitted infections (STIs) are primarily a concern for younger people, making safe sex seem unnecessary for older adults. This misunderstanding can lead to real risks, as older adults who remain sexually active are still susceptible to STIs. Unfortunately, this myth often leaves older adults unaware or under-informed about protecting their sexual health, and some may feel uncomfortable discussing sexual health openly. By understanding that sexual health is important at every age, you can confidently take steps to stay safe, informed, and proactive about your well-being.

STI-Real Talk

It's essential to update your understanding of sexual health terminology. The term "sexually transmitted diseases" (STDs) is no longer entirely accurate, as not all sexually transmitted conditions are classified as diseases. Some are infections, such as syphilis, gonorrhea, chlamydia, and trichomoniasis—which are bacterial infections that can be cured with proper treatment.

Viral infections like hepatitis B, herpes simplex virus (HSV), human papillomavirus (HPV), and HIV/AIDS are persistent. They cannot be cured but can be managed with appropriate medical care.

Among U.S. adults aged 65 and older, STI rates more than doubled between 2012 and 2020. Rates of syphilis, chlamydia, gonorrhea, herpes, HPV, and HIV/AIDS are all on the rise and are expected to continue climbing as the aging population grows. This increase is partly due to a lack of awareness and education about sexual health among this age group.

In The Villages, 19% of men and 11% of women reported having experienced a sexually transmitted infection (STI) at some point in their lives. When asked about safe practices with new partners, 86% of women reported they would prioritize protection. In contrast, 61% of men admitted they would likely forgo using a condom.

These statistics reveal a noticeable difference in how men and women approach sexual health and protection—while most women are focused on staying safe with new partners, many men are more likely to skip protection. This highlights the need for more open conversations and awareness about safe sex for everyone.

Rising STI rates among older adults underscore the need for better awareness and education about sexual health, particularly in communities where intimacy remains an important part of life. Open conversations with healthcare providers about STI prevention, condom use, and sexual wellness can help you enjoy healthy relationships with peace of mind. Let's ensure that your approach to sexual health is as vibrant and active as your lifestyle!

Case History: Harry's Poolside Revelation

Among the intriguing characters of The Villages, I met Harry—a charming and humorous man who became a friend during my regular visits to the pool. Harry was known for cracking jokes to anyone within earshot. He had an infectious laugh and a knack for storytelling.

One day, between laps and laughter, Harry confided in me about an embarrassing development. "I've got herpes," he said with a sigh, quickly followed by, "Guess retirement isn't as dull as I thought it'd be!"

Harry's revelation was as unexpected as it was enlightening. He recounted how he met a lovely lady at one of the many social events. "We hit it off instantly," he said with a grin. But a few weeks later, he started experiencing some uncomfortable symptoms. "Let's just say it wasn't the kind of burning desire I'd hoped for," he quipped. A visit to the doctor confirmed it.

Harry faced his diagnosis with a mix of humor and practicality. "Well, at least it's not fatal," he joked, "Just really inconvenient." He educated himself on managing the condition, understanding the importance of medication, and the need for open communication with future partners. "I had to brush up on my birds and bees talk," he laughed, "Who knew I'd be having the 'safe sex' talk again at my age?"

Despite the initial shock and embarrassment, Harry found solace in humor and support from friends. He was open about his condition, using it as an opportunity to educate others about safe sex practices. "It's not the end of the world," he'd say, "Just a reminder to always play it safe." His openness sparked many candid conversations poolside, making everyone more aware and less judgmental.

Key Lessons:

- **Use Humor to Cope:** Harry approached his herpes diagnosis with humor, which helped ease the discomfort around a sensitive topic. His ability to laugh at his situation made it easier for himself and others to engage in open discussions.

- **Educate and Share Knowledge:** After learning how to manage herpes, Harry took the initiative to educate others about his condition. By sharing his experience, he promoted awareness and safe sex practices, turning a personal challenge into an opportunity to inform others.

- **Foster Open Communication:** Harry's willingness to talk openly about his diagnosis encouraged honest conversations with his friends. His transparency helped reduce stigma and created a more understanding and supportive environment.

Playing It Safe

Practicing safe sex is essential for preventing sexually transmitted infections (STIs) and maintaining your sexual health. Using condoms and other barrier methods can protect you and your partner from infections, ensuring that your sexual experiences are safe and worry-free. Regular STI screenings and open communication with your partner are critical steps in maintaining safety. Educating yourself about safe sex practices and being proactive in protecting your health leads to a more confident and enjoyable sex life. Prioritizing safe practices shows respect for your health and your partner's, fostering a responsible and healthy approach to intimacy.

Health Checks That Matter

Living in The Villages brings unique challenges for maintaining sexual health and well-being. Age-related changes, the risk of STIs, and persistent stigmas around aging and sexuality can sometimes complicate things. However, regular sexual health screenings and check-ups are essential to managing these complexities. These visits allow your healthcare provider to address any concerns directly, whether it's adjusting medications or exploring 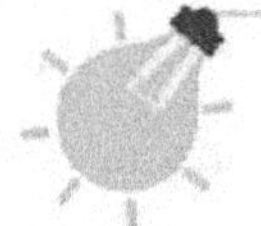

hormone replacement therapy (HRT). By making health check-ups a priority, you can confidently overcome age-related hurdles and continue to enjoy a fulfilling, healthy intimate life.

Sexual health screenings should be a regular part of your care. Your healthcare provider should routinely conduct comprehensive sexual health assessments to keep things running smoothly and help you make informed decisions about safe sex practices, STI prevention, and other sexual health issues. These assessments look at your sexual history (including STIs/HIV), medication use, sexual functioning, and any behaviors that might pose health risks.

A comprehensive sexual assessment should incorporate your sexual orientation and gender identity (SOGI). Gathering SOGI information enables healthcare providers to address issues contributing to disparities experienced by lesbian, gay, bisexual, transgender, queer, and other sexual minority (LGBTQ+) populations. This data is crucial for advancing sexual health equality to ensure all people receive informed and inclusive care.

Barriers Exposed

Many older adults feel they miss out on meaningful conversations about sexual health with their doctors. Research shows that healthcare providers often overlook this crucial aspect of care, particularly among older patients. In one study of 500 doctors treating patients aged 50 and older, only 2% said they routinely ask about their patients' sexual health. Another study found that just 38% of male patients and 22% of female patients discussed sexual health with their primary care doctors—with 61% rarely or never addressing STIs. Additionally, 78% of patients with erectile dysfunction (ED) hadn't discussed the issue with their doctors, even though 82% wished their doctor had brought up the topic to ease their embarrassment.

Many sexual health issues go unaddressed for a range of reasons. Often, healthcare providers aren't given adequate training or may feel uneasy bringing up these sensitive topics. Pressing time limits, patient privacy concerns, and the difficulty of navigating delicate conversations add to the challenge. Other obstacles include mismatches in age or gender between providers and patients, limited support systems, and outdated electronic health record (EHR) systems that fail to prioritize sexual health.

For younger or less experienced healthcare providers, talking about sexual health with older patients can feel especially daunting. Even in open-minded communities, like The Villages—stigma around topics like sexual health, sexual orientation, and aging may hold residents back from getting the care they need.

Closing this gap requires commitment from both patients and healthcare providers to place sexual health higher on their list of priorities. It starts with open, supportive communication and an understanding that sexual wellness is a crucial part of overall health.

Here are some steps you can take:

- **Be Proactive:** Don't hesitate to bring up your sexual health concerns during your medical appointments. Your well-being is essential, and your doctor is there to help.

- **Ask Questions:** If your doctor doesn't ask about your sexual health, bring it up yourself. Ask about preventing STIs, safe sex practices, and any other concerns regarding sexual functioning.

- **Educate Yourself:** Look for reliable information about sexual health. Being informed will help you have better discussions with your healthcare provider.

- **Encourage a Supportive Environment:** Help your doctor create a supportive atmosphere where you feel comfortable discussing intimate topics.

- **Advocate for Comprehensive Care:** Ensure your care includes regular sexual health assessments. This will ensure that any issues are addressed promptly and effectively.

Sex Ed for Grown-Ups

Taking charge of your sexual health is essential to living a confident, fulfilling life. Staying informed on the latest insights, treatments, and strategies keeps intimacy enjoyable and enhances your overall well-being. There are countless ways to stay educated—reading reliable books, browsing trustworthy websites, attending local workshops, or joining supportive groups—each option giving you tools to build a healthier, more satisfying intimate life.

In The Villages, you have access to a wealth of resources designed to support your sexual wellness. This dynamic community offers educational seminars, workshops, and personalized counseling, empowering you to make informed choices. You're encouraged to prioritize your health by exploring safe sexual practices, seeking regular STI screenings, and engaging with available resources.

Living a healthy, intimate life in your later years should feel rewarding and worry-free. By using the support and services at your fingertips, you can stay proactive, confident, and ready to embrace each new day.

Tips:

- **Empower Yourself with Knowledge:** Don't let myths and stereotypes hold you back—get the facts and stay informed about the sexual health screenings you need. Understanding the current information about sexual health gives you the power to keep your intimate life exciting and safe.

- **Stay Informed:** Always put your health first by practicing safe sex and using protection to prevent STIs if you're sexually active. Regular check-ups and sexual health screenings are crucial for catching potential issues early to maintain your health and well-being.

CHAPTER 4

Sex Stats

"The age of a woman doesn't mean a thing. The best tunes are played on the oldest fiddles."

— Ralph Waldo Emerson, American Philosopher

What The Research Says

As people live longer and Baby Boomers age, the number of older adults is rapidly increasing. In 2021, about 1 in 6 people in the U.S. were aged 65 or older, making up 16% of the population. By 2030, adults over 65 years of age are expected to make up 20% of the global population. This change enhances the importance of understanding the factors that contribute to the well-being of older adults.

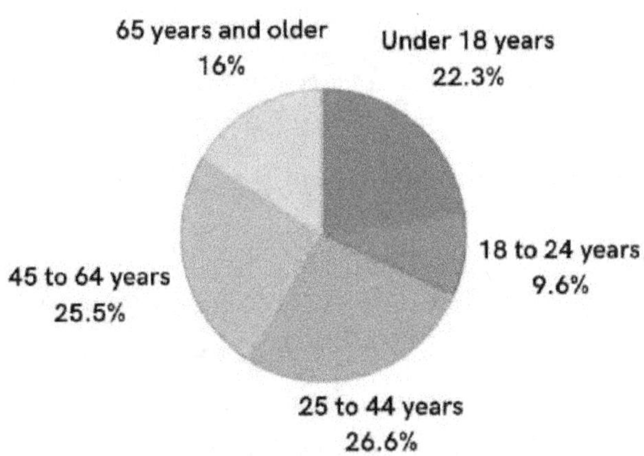

Despite the progress made in understanding human sexuality, the sexual health of older adults is often overlooked, even in active, independent retirement communities like The Villages. While much research has been done on sexual behavior across various age groups, the unique needs, concerns, and challenges you may face as an older adult are too frequently neglected.

But your later years are a time to embrace joy, intimacy, and connection—experiences that can bring greater meaning and richness to your life. Prioritizing your sexual health is about more than just physical well-being; it's about nurturing emotional closeness, self-confidence, and personal fulfillment.

By focusing on this often-ignored aspect of wellness, you help create a community that values all dimensions of health, including sexual health. When sexual health is acknowledged and supported as an integral part of life, it fosters an environment where everyone's well-being is truly honored. You deserve to enjoy every part of life, including a vibrant, satisfying, intimate connection that enhances your overall quality of life.

Sex and The Happy Factor

Does sex make you happy? Research says yes! Studies of older adults in the U.S. show a strong link between sexual activity and happiness. Some studies even suggest that regular sexual activity can bring more joy and happiness than an increase in income. Those in good health reported greater sexual satisfaction compared to their less sprightly counterparts.

Research also shows that passion doesn't fade with age. Many older adults continue to enjoy an active sex life well into their later years. According to the National Social Life, Health, and Aging Project, a significant number of older adults remain sexually active. About 73% of people aged 57-64, 53% of those aged 65-74, and 26% of adults aged 75-85 report being sexually active.

Percentage of Older Adults Who Are Sexually Active

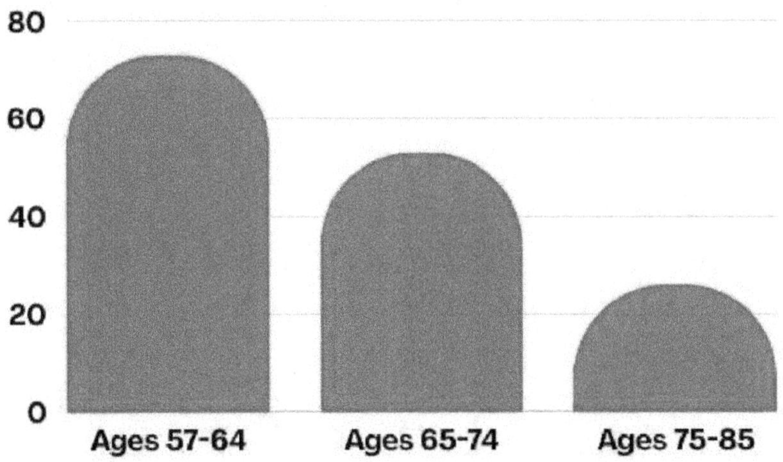

Sexual health remains a key factor in the overall well-being of many older adults. One U.S. study found that 62% of men and 43% of women say it plays a crucial role in their quality of life. What's particularly interesting is that men often show that age doesn't stand in the way of keeping an active and fulfilling sex life. Let's take a closer look at how residents of The Villages embrace intimacy as they age.

Data from The Villages shows that many residents keep their romantic lives active well into their later years. In fact, 62% of those surveyed reported current engagement in sexual activities. Notably, 66% of women and 79% of men believe that staying sexually active is important for maintaining a healthy and satisfying relationship. These insights highlight the fact that for many residents, intimacy remains a vital part of life as they grow older.

Generations and Their Views

Generations like Baby Boomers (1946-1964) and Gen X (1965-1980) have been deeply influenced by the major events and cultural changes of their youth. Important moments like the Civil Rights Movement, the Sexual Revolution, the Women's Liberation Movement, and technological advances have significantly shaped their beliefs and behaviors. These experiences have left a lasting impact on how each generation views the world and interacts with it.

In the past, views on aging and sexuality were quite different. Sigmund Freud believed that sexual desire naturally declined with age, particularly for women after menopause. Many women saw sex as a duty to their husbands, often without experiencing much sexual satisfaction themselves. However, modern research challenges Freud's outdated beliefs, revealing that sexuality remains a complex and vital part of life, evolving but not disappearing with age.

Baby Boomers, in particular, have a different outlook on sexuality compared to previous generations. As leaders of the Sexual Revolution, they continue to challenge outdated norms and beliefs. While some taboos around sex and aging still exist, Baby Boomers are showing that desire doesn't fade with age—it changes and can bring new opportunities for connection and pleasure.

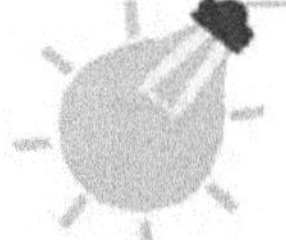

Older adults who maintain an active sex life report higher levels of overall happiness and life satisfaction

Pills, Potions, and Passion

Baby Boomers have turned challenges into opportunities, thanks to medications that enhance sexual performance. Drugs like Viagra have made it possible for older adults to enjoy sexual activities that used to seem out of reach. With more open discussions about aging and sexuality, this generation is now able to embrace their desires without feeling guilty or ashamed.

These medications address physical challenges that come with age and combined with open discussions with healthcare providers, have reduced many of the taboos surrounding sex in later life. This openness has led to better sexual health care for older adults, including regular check-ups and honest conversations with doctors. Baby Boomers are also setting an example for younger generations by showing that sexuality is a lifelong journey. Their proactive approach to health and open attitudes about their sexual lives are helping to create a more inclusive view of aging and sexuality.

Redefining Relationships

As Baby Boomers move into their sixties, seventies, and beyond, they continue challenging and reshaping traditional views on love, intimacy, and partnership. Just as they pioneered social change during the Sexual Revolution, this generation now pushes against old notions of what relationships should look like in later life. Many Baby Boomers are opting for "gray divorces"—a rising trend of late-life separations—highlighting their commitment to personal happiness and fulfillment at every stage of life.

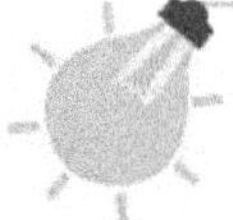

DID YOU KNOW?

Residents of The Villages report having a more active sex life than the national average for their age group

Many of you are seeking relationships that bring joy, satisfaction, and authenticity. Whether through rekindling connections with long-term partners or forming new relationships, Baby Boomers are proving that love and intimacy are dynamic, evolving parts of life. The desire for fulfilling relationships demonstrates that contentment is not something to be sacrificed for tradition or longevity. Instead, it is a central goal, one that is reshaping societal expectations of aging and companionship.

According to the Pew Research Center, the divorce rate for Americans over 50 has doubled since the 1990s. This newfound freedom from long-term marriages often leads to a renaissance of romance and sexual exploration. Many are now embracing fluidity, independence, and authenticity in their partnerships. From second marriages to non-traditional arrangements, many Baby Boomers are charting new territories of love and companionship. However, these relationship shifts also bring challenges, such as navigating blended families, empty nest syndrome, and the complexities of starting anew in later life.

While some of you are diving headfirst into new romantic and sexual adventures, others are redefining what intimacy means. For many, companionship and emotional connection have taken precedence over physical romance.

This shift reveals a growing recognition of the deep fulfillment that platonic relationships can offer, particularly in reducing stress, promoting mental well-being, and enhancing overall health. In this stage of life, close friendships and emotional bonds are becoming as valuable as romantic partnerships, showing that intimacy is about connection, not just sexuality.

Baby Boomers remind us that love, relationships, and intimacy don't fade with age—they evolve. The desire for meaningful connections remains strong, and how these connections are formed and valued continues to redefine how society views aging, love, and happiness.

Tips:

- **Embrace Change and Redefine Your Path:** Life's transitions, such as losing a partner, divorce, or embarking on new beginnings, can reshape your relationships and sense of identity. Instead of fearing these changes, approach them as opportunities for self-exploration and growth. Allow yourself to evolve, rediscover your strengths, and redefine what relationships mean in this new chapter of life. This adaptation process can lead to deeper self-awareness and a more fulfilling connection with others.

- **Welcome New Perspectives for Emotional Growth:** Emotional transitions can feel overwhelming, but they also offer a chance to invite fresh perspectives and build meaningful connections. By remaining open to new relationships, experiences, and ideas, you create space for emotional and mental growth. These connections not only provide support but can also inspire a renewed sense of purpose. During challenging times, actively seek new conversations and experiences that push you beyond your comfort zone. It's in these moments of openness that your resilience and personal growth will truly flourish.

CHAPTER 5

Problems In Paradise

"Sex at age 90 is like trying to shoot pool with a rope."
— George Burns, American Comedian

Sexual Health Woes

As you age, your sexual health may go through noticeable changes, with sexual dysfunction becoming more common for both men and women. These challenges can stem from various factors, including shifts in your body's hormones, chronic health conditions, medications, and emotional well-being—all evolving over time. Hormonal changes, illness, and even stress can influence your sexual experiences as you get older. Understanding why sexual dysfunction occurs and knowing the available treatments can help you maintain strong relationships and encourage open conversations about intimacy.

For men, testosterone levels start to decline around age 30, dropping about 1% each year. This can affect libido and lead to erectile dysfunction (ED). As testosterone decreases, sperm production also falls, and ED may become more common. Factors like reduced blood flow, nerve sensitivity, and low hormone levels can contribute to these issues. It's essential to consult a healthcare provider if you're experiencing ED. Treatments and lifestyle changes such as maintaining a healthy weight, avoiding smoking, and limiting alcohol can help improve erectile function.

For women, menopause can significantly affect sexual function. Menopause typically begins in the late 40s to early 50s, causing a drop in estrogen levels that can lower libido and lead to hypoactive sexual desire disorder (HSDD). Sexual dysfunction is more common in women than in men. The decline in estrogen can cause vaginal dryness and discomfort during sex. However, hormone therapy, along with lubricants and moisturizers, can help alleviate these symptoms and enhance sexual function. Staying mindful of how aging impacts your sexual health and taking proactive measures to address those changes can go a long way in keeping the passion alive and maintaining intimacy throughout your life!

Chronic Illness and Bedroom Blues

Chronic diseases are widespread and can significantly affect your sexual health, often leading to challenges in intimacy and well-being. Additionally, they place a more significant burden on healthcare systems, highlighting the importance of managing these conditions effectively. Conditions like diabetes, heart disease, and hypertension can affect your body's ability to function sexually, lowering your quality of life. However, many of these diseases can be prevented by making healthier choices. Eating well, exercising regularly, and maintaining a healthy weight can reduce the risk of chronic illness and help you maintain your sexual health as you age. These lifestyle changes support your overall well-being and help you stay more active and fulfilled in your intimate relationships. Taking control of your health now can lead to a healthier, more satisfying life in the future.

Staying healthy isn't just about adding years to your life—it's about enhancing your quality of life and enjoying every moment to its fullest. Maintaining optimal health allows you to remain physically and emotionally active, engaged, and vibrant. In The Villages, many residents face chronic health conditions that not only affect overall wellness but can also influence sexual function. Next, we'll explore the seven most common chronic conditions affecting older adults, along with practical management strategies, medications commonly prescribed, and how these factors can impact sexual health. By understanding and addressing these issues, you can take proactive steps to maintain your health and sexual well-being.

High Cholesterol

High cholesterol can directly affect sexual health by limiting blood flow, not just to the heart but also to the genitals. This reduced circulation can contribute to issues such as erectile dysfunction (ED) in men and decreased arousal or lubrication in women. The plaque buildup in arteries, a result of high cholesterol, can make it difficult to achieve or maintain an erection and may also impair sexual performance and satisfaction. Over time, these effects can diminish intimacy and overall well-being, emphasizing the importance of managing cholesterol levels for cardiovascular and sexual health.

Managing cholesterol through lifestyle changes is critical to maintaining sexual health. A diet rich in heart-healthy foods, such as vegetables, fruits, whole grains, and healthy fats, can help reduce cholesterol levels and improve circulation. Regular aerobic exercises like walking, cycling, or swimming can boost cardiovascular health and enhance libido and sexual performance.

In many cases, medications such as statins are prescribed to manage cholesterol levels, and by improving circulation, these treatments can also enhance sexual health. By addressing high cholesterol early, individuals can boost cardiovascular function and maintain or restore sexual vitality. Proactively managing cholesterol is key to supporting heart health and a fulfilling sex life.

High Blood Pressure

High blood pressure, or hypertension, can have a profound effect on sexual health, often causing difficulties with arousal and sexual performance. In men, hypertension can lead to ED by limiting blood flow. In women, it may cause a decrease in libido, reduced vaginal lubrication, or difficulty achieving orgasm.

Lifestyle changes can significantly improve blood pressure levels and sexual health. Reducing sodium intake, avoiding processed foods, and focusing on a diet rich in fruits, vegetables, and lean proteins can help lower blood pressure and support healthy circulation. Regular physical activity helps manage blood pressure, increase stamina, improve mood, and boost sexual function. Managing stress is also crucial, as chronic stress can raise blood pressure and decrease sexual desire. Relaxation techniques like deep breathing, meditation, or yoga can help control stress and enhance well-being.

Medications such as beta-blockers or diuretics may be necessary to manage high blood pressure. Still, it's important to discuss any potential side effects with your doctor, as some medications can affect sexual performance. Addressing high blood pressure through medical treatments and lifestyle changes can improve your heart health, leading to a more fulfilling and satisfying intimate life.

Arthritis

Joint pain can dampen your intimacy, making certain positions uncomfortable or challenging. Maintaining a healthy weight alleviates joint pressure and reduces arthritis symptoms. Low-impact exercises like swimming, cycling, yoga, or tai chi can enhance joint mobility and relieve pain.

Medications like NSAIDs (ibuprofen and naproxen), corticosteroids, DMARDs, and biologics play a crucial role in managing arthritis symptoms. It's important to recognize that corticosteroids, particularly with long-term use, have been linked to reduced libido and overall sexual desire. Additionally, the chronic pain associated with arthritis can further diminish sex drive. However, exploring comfortable positions and implementing effective pain management strategies can help alleviate discomfort and maintain intimacy.

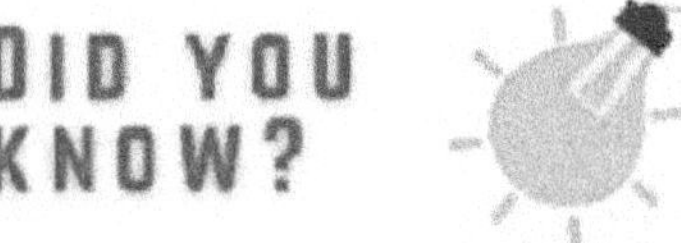

An active sex life can strengthen the immune system, helping to ward off common illnesses

Heart Conditions

Heart conditions can sometimes take a toll on your sex life, leaving you feeling out of breath or hesitant to engage in more physical activities. However, you can still enjoy a fulfilling love life by managing your heart health. Start by following a heart-healthy diet, like the DASH plan, which focuses on plenty of fruits, vegetables, whole grains, and low-fat dairy while limiting sodium. Staying active with regular exercise is also key to keeping your heart strong.

Common medications for heart conditions include beta-blockers (like atenolol and metoprolol), diuretics, ACE inhibitors (like lisinopril), and calcium channel blockers (like amlodipine). While beta-blockers and diuretics can sometimes lead to sexual side effects, such as reduced libido or erectile difficulties, ACE inhibitors and calcium channel blockers are less likely to affect your sexual health.

Diabetes

This metabolic mischief-maker can wreak havoc on your sexual function, causing nerve damage, decreased sensation, reduced blood flow, and erectile difficulties. Managing diabetes requires a strategic approach to keep blood sugar levels under control. It is important to monitor your blood sugar levels regularly and follow a diabetes-friendly diet that balances carbohydrates, proteins, and healthy fats.

Medications to treat diabetes include insulin, metformin, sulfonylureas (glipizide), thiazolidinediones (pioglitazone), or other injectable options. Some medications have been linked to lower testosterone levels, potentially impacting libido and sexual desire.

Depression

Depression can significantly dampen your sexual desire and disrupt pleasure in your intimate relationships. Regular exercise, balanced nutrition, stress management techniques, and social support can help alleviate symptoms.

Therapy, such as cognitive-behavioral therapy (CBT) or interpersonal therapy (IPT) can address underlying issues, while medications like SSRIs, SNRIs, TCAs, and MAOIs work to rebalance brain chemicals. These medications may have sexual side effects, including decreased libido and ED. Combining lifestyle changes, therapy, and careful medication management can help restore sexual intimacy.

Nervous Conditions

From anxiety to neurological disorders, nervous system issues can throw a wrench in your gears of sexual response, making it challenging to achieve arousal or orgasm. Stress management techniques, regular exercise, adequate sleep, and a nutritious diet support nervous system function. Therapy, such as CBT or exposure therapy, provides valuable tools for effectively managing symptoms.

Medications like benzodiazepines (diazepam and lorazepam), SSRIs, SNRIs, and buspirone are commonly prescribed. Benzodiazepines can decrease libido, while SSRIs and SNRIs can significantly impact sexual function. Buspirone, however, has been shown to have fewer sexual side effects.

Managing Medications

Effectively managing your medications can help ensure you take the correct dose at the right time, which is crucial for maintaining health. One of the simplest ways to stay organized is by using a pill organizer, which allows you to sort your medications by day and time. Setting alarms or reminders on your phone or smartwatch can be a great way to ensure you never miss a dose, especially for medications that need to be taken at specific intervals. There are also medication management apps that provide alerts and track your intake. Additionally, keeping a medication log or checklist can help you monitor when and how much medication you've taken, reducing the risk of missing a dose or accidentally doubling up. Consider consulting your pharmacist or doctor to create a simplified medication schedule if you're managing multiple medications.

Case History: Steve's Swing at Life

Among the vibrant crowd at The Villages, I had the pleasure of befriending Steve, a jovial golfer from Michigan. We met on the golf course, where his infectious banter and impressive swing quickly made him a favorite in our group.

One day, after sinking a particularly tricky putt, Steve turned to us with a serious expression and said, "I've got some news that's harder to manage than my golf handicap—I've been diagnosed with MS." His candidness and resilience left a lasting impression on all of us.

Steve noticed something was amiss when he began experiencing numbness in his hands and legs. "At first, I thought it was just my body's way of telling me to stop missing putts," he joked. After a series of doctor visits and tests, the diagnosis was precise: Steve had Multiple Sclerosis.

Steve faced his diagnosis with the same determination he applied to his golf game. "MS might mess with my body, but it won't mess with my spirit," he declared. He adjusted his routine, incorporating regular physiotherapy and ensuring enough rest. But the challenges of MS didn't stop at mobility—they extended into the bedroom.

Steve was candid about how MS affected his sexual health. "It's like my body decided to play a cruel joke," he said, "because if dealing with numb legs wasn't enough, now my libido needs a pep talk." He sought medical advice and explored treatments to manage this aspect of his condition. "Turns out, talking to your doctor about sex is less awkward than shanking a ball into the neighbor's yard," he laughed.

Despite the challenges, Steve's humor remained intact. He often joked, "If I can get through a round of golf with these symptoms, I can get through anything." His openness about his condition and its impact on his life, including his sexual health, made it easier for others to discuss their struggles. His positive outlook and openness were both comforting and inspiring.

Key Lessons:

- **Face Challenges with Humor and Positivity:** Steve approached his MS diagnosis with humor and determination, keeping his spirit strong despite physical challenges. This emphasizes the value of maintaining a positive outlook during difficult times.

- **Adapt to Health Changes:** Steve made lifestyle adjustments, like regular physiotherapy and sufficient rest, to manage his condition. His proactive approach highlights the importance of adapting and managing chronic illnesses to maintain a high quality of life.

- **Communicate About Health and Intimacy:** Steve openly discussed how MS affected his sexual health and sought medical advice to address his issues. His transparency highlights the importance of honest communication about health issues and their positive impact on relationships.

Sex for a Long Life

Did you know? Sex can help you live longer! That's right—keeping an active sex life as you age brings many benefits that can significantly enhance your longevity and quality of life. Studies show that sex improves your physical, mental, and emotional well-being. Here are twelve proven ways regular sexual activity helps you live longer:

1. **Improves Heart Health:** Regular sex is good for your heart. It helps lower blood pressure, improves circulation, and reduces the risk of heart disease. Think of it as a fun form of exercise that benefits your heart.

2. **Boosts Your Immune System:** Engaging in sex increases the production of antibodies, which help your body fight off infections and illnesses. This means you're less likely to get sick and more likely to stay healthy.

3. **Reduces Stress:** Sex triggers the release of hormones like endorphins and oxytocin. These hormones help reduce stress and create happiness and relaxation, improving overall health.

4. **Improves Sleep Quality:** The hormones released during sex, such as oxytocin and prolactin, promote relaxation and help you fall asleep faster. And better sleep leads to better health.

5. **Increases Longevity:** Studies show that people who have sex regularly tend to live longer. Combining physical exercise, emotional bonding, and stress reduction contributes to a longer lifespan.

6. **Enhances Emotional Well-being:** Being intimate with someone helps build emotional connections, reducing feelings of loneliness and

depression. A solid emotional bond leads to a happier and more fulfilling life.

7. **Balances Hormones:** Sex helps regulate hormone levels, including important ones like testosterone and estrogen. Balanced hormones are crucial for maintaining overall health, especially as you age.

8. **Boosts Brain Health:** Regular sexual activity can improve cognitive function and memory. It increases blood flow to the brain and promotes the growth of new brain cells, keeping your mind sharp. So, does sex make you smarter? It just might!

9. **Provides Pain Relief:** The endorphins released during sex act as natural painkillers. They can help alleviate chronic pain conditions such as arthritis and migraines, providing much-needed relief.

10. **Increases Self-esteem:** A healthy sex life can boost your self-esteem and confidence. Feeling good about yourself and your relationships is essential for your mental health and happiness.

11. **Strengthens Relationships:** Sexual intimacy strengthens the bond between partners. A strong, supportive relationship contributes to emotional stability and overall well-being, which are linked to a longer life.

12. **Promotes Physical Fitness:** Staying physically active is vital to maintaining optimal health and longevity—and sex is a form of physical exercise. It helps burn calories, improve muscle tone, and increase flexibility.

Tips:

- **Manage Your Chronic Health Conditions:** Take control of your health by following your treatment plans and making necessary lifestyle changes. Managing chronic conditions like diabetes, heart disease, or arthritis can improve your ability to enjoy intimate moments with your partner and keep your love life thriving.

- **Keep an Eye on Your Medications**: Some medications can impact your sexual health. If you notice side effects, talk to your healthcare provider. They may be able to adjust your treatment or suggest alternatives that support both your health and sexual well-being.

CHAPTER 6

Fueling the Fire

"If music be the food of love, play on."
— William Shakespeare, English Playwright

Food for the Mood

Nutrition is essential for maintaining sexual health and overall vitality. Just as food fuels your body, food impacts your sex drive and performance. Certain foods can enhance sexual function, leading to longer-lasting erections, better lubrication, and more intense orgasms.

Your diet also affects your mood and stress levels. Foods rich in tryptophan, like turkey and bananas, boost serotonin levels, which promote relaxation and well-being. A well-rounded diet with essential nutrients—vitamins, minerals, antioxidants, and healthy fats—supports overall health, balances hormones, and ensures proper blood circulation, all important for optimal sexual function.

On the other hand, poor dietary choices are harmful. Diets high in saturated fats, trans fats, salt, and processed foods can lead to atherosclerosis and cardiovascular diseases. These health conditions can hinder blood flow and result in erectile dysfunction (ED) and reduced libido. Excessive caffeine, alcohol, or refined sugars can affect your mood and increase stress, lowering sexual desire. Heavy, greasy foods can make you feel sluggish rather than energetic. Moreover, being overweight can cause hormonal imbalances, lower testosterone levels, and increase the risk of diabetes and hypertension.

Making healthier food choices can support your overall health and lead to a more fulfilling sex life.

Beneficial Dietary Patterns

A well-balanced diet plays a significant role in maintaining sexual health and vitality. Certain dietary patterns, such as the Mediterranean Diet and the DASH Diet, have been shown to offer specific benefits that support cardiovascular health. These diets emphasize nutrient-rich, whole foods that improve physical health and positively impact sexual function. By promoting heart health, regulating blood pressure, and providing essential nutrients, these dietary approaches offer a natural and effective way to support overall health. Maintaining a healthy weight through balanced eating can help prevent chronic conditions, which are often linked to sexual dysfunction. By nourishing both the body and mind, a well-rounded diet can enhance not only overall wellness but also sexual satisfaction and intimacy.

The Mediterranean Diet: This diet emphasizes whole grains, fruits, vegetables, legumes, nuts, and olive oil, with moderate portions of fish and poultry. It is rich in antioxidants, healthy fats, and fiber, supporting cardiovascular health and sexual function. It promotes whole, natural foods and a balanced lifestyle.

The DASH Diet: The Dietary Approaches to Stop Hypertension (DASH) diet focuses on reducing sodium intake and increasing potassium-rich foods like fruits and vegetables. This helps regulate blood pressure, which is crucial for maintaining erectile function and overall sexual health.

Hydration for Vitality

Staying hydrated is crucial for your sexual health and well-being, especially as you age. In sunny places like The Villages, where the heat can be intense, staying well-hydrated is even more critical. Proper hydration helps regulate your body temperature, reducing the risk of heat-related issues like exhaustion and heatstroke, which can impact your energy levels and desire. Staying well hydrated is essential for supporting your immune system, which is key in defending your body against infections and illnesses that can negatively impact your sex life.

Drinking enough water helps flush out toxins, keeps your organs functioning optimally, and ensures that your cells are well-nourished and ready to combat potential threats. Adequate hydration also improves blood circulation, which

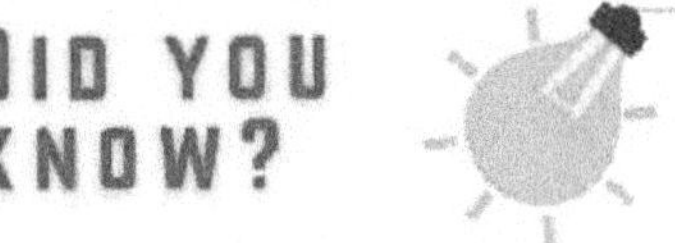

Staying hydrated is essential for maintaining sexual health, as dehydration can lead to fatigue and decreased libido

is vital for sexual health, as it enhances arousal and performance by promoting better oxygen flow to tissues. In addition, hydration aids in maintaining energy levels, reducing fatigue, and balancing hormones, all of which are critical for a healthy and fulfilling intimate life.

Your metabolism naturally slows down as you age, making weight gain easier. Mindful eating can be a powerful tool to manage this change. You can maintain a healthier weight by paying attention to your body's hunger signals, using smaller plates, and avoiding overeating. Choosing nutritious foods boosts your mood, reduces stress, and promotes optimal sexual function, helping you enjoy a satisfying and vibrant love life. Staying hydrated and maintaining a balanced diet can support your sexual well-being and satisfaction.

Power of Nutrients

Nutrients are essential for growth, development, and the maintenance of life, ensuring that every system in the body functions optimally. Regarding sexual health, the role of nutrients becomes even more critical. Macronutrients—proteins, fats, and carbohydrates—provide the energy and structural building blocks needed to support hormonal balance, stamina, and reproductive function. Micronutrients—vitamins and minerals—are equally important, working behind the scenes to regulate everything from blood flow to nerve function.

Each nutrient, whether it's a protein essential for muscle repair or a mineral vital for maintaining energy levels, plays a distinct and crucial role in keeping your body—and your sex life—running smoothly. Nutrients are categorized into macronutrients and micronutrients. Macronutrients and micronutrients are crucial for your sexual well-being and overall health.

Macronutrients for Passion

Macronutrients, including carbohydrates, proteins, and fats, are essential nutrients required in large quantities to sustain key bodily functions. A well-balanced intake of these macronutrients fuels the body with energy and provides the structural components and hormonal support necessary for optimal physical, mental, and sexual health.

Carbohydrates: Essential Energy Providers

Carbohydrates are the primary energy source for your body and are essential for all activity. Maintaining energy levels becomes crucial for overall vitality and health as you age. Carbohydrates help boost energy, enhance mood, and stabilize blood sugar levels. Key sources include:

Whole Grains: Whole grains provide sustained energy by slowly releasing glucose into the bloodstream. This helps you maintain stamina and avoid energy slumps during activity. Examples include oats, quinoa, brown rice, barley, and whole wheat.

Fruits: Fruits are rich in vitamins, antioxidants, and fiber. They boost energy levels, enhance mood, and improve overall health. Examples include berries, bananas, apples, and citrus fruits.

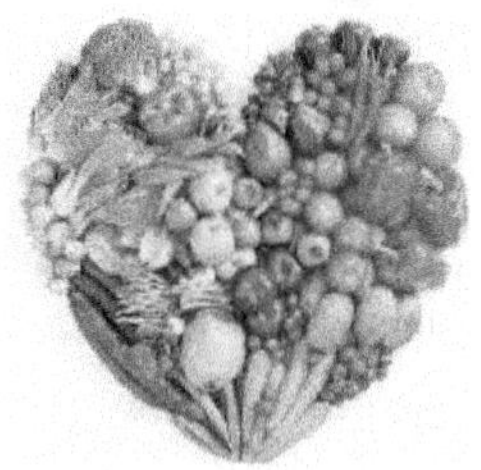

Vegetables: Vegetables supply essential nutrients and complex carbohydrates to support overall health and energy. Examples are sweet potatoes, carrots, spinach, and kale.

Legumes: High in fiber and complex carbohydrates, legumes provide steady energy and support digestive health. Examples include lentils, chickpeas, black beans, and kidney beans.

Proteins: Builders and Repairers

Proteins are crucial for building and repairing tissues, producing enzymes and hormones, and supporting the immune system. Adequate protein intake is essential for maintaining muscle mass, hormone balance, and overall health. Key sources include:

Lean Meats: Lean meats are rich in protein and essential amino acids, supporting muscle maintenance, hormone production, and overall physical strength needed for sexual activity. Examples include chicken, turkey, and lean cuts of beef.

Fish: Fatty fish, especially salmon, mackerel, sardines, and trout, are high in omega-3 fatty acids. These acids enhance blood flow and support cardiovascular health.

Eggs: Eggs are a complete protein source, providing all essential amino acids. They also contain vitamins B6 and B5, which help balance hormone levels and reduce stress—contributing to greater health and well-being.

Nuts and Seeds: Nuts and seeds are high in protein, healthy fats, and essential vitamins and minerals. They boost energy levels, improve blood flow, and support hormone production. Examples are almonds, walnuts, chia seeds, and flaxseeds.

Fats: Energy Storage and Protectors

Fats play several bodily roles, including storing energy, insulating and protecting organs, and producing sex hormones. They also help absorb fat-soluble vitamins. Key sources include:

Omega-3 Fatty Acids: These essential fats are renowned for boosting heart health and improving circulation, which are crucial for peak sexual performance and stamina. Omega-3s are also fantastic for reducing inflammation and supporting brain health. You'll find these healthy fats in fatty fish, such as salmon, mackerel, and sardines, as well as in flaxseeds, chia seeds, and walnuts.

Monounsaturated Fats: These healthy fats help maintain cholesterol levels and improve heart health, which is crucial for sexual function and endurance. You can find these in olive oil, avocados, nuts (like almonds, hazelnuts, and pecans), and seeds (such as pumpkin and sesame seeds).

Polyunsaturated Fats: Omega-6 fatty acids are essential for hormone production and cell membrane integrity. They are found in sunflower, corn, soybean, and fatty fish oils.

Saturated Fats (in moderation): These fats play a role in hormone production and cellular function. However, excessive intake can lead to clogged arteries and reduced blood flow, potentially impacting sexual performance. Foods containing saturated fats include butter, cheese, red meat, and coconut oil.

Micronutrients for Longevity

Micronutrients, including essential vitamins and minerals, are critical for maintaining overall health. Their role in promoting longevity has been extensively studied, showing that these nutrients support vital bodily functions, protect against chronic diseases, and enhance energy levels. What's less discussed, however, is how they directly impact sexual health. Optimal levels of key micronutrients contribute to hormone balance, reproductive function, and libido—all essential for sustaining a healthy and fulfilling intimate life.

Vitamins for Libido

Vitamins are crucial for maintaining a healthy and active sex life, although their importance is often overlooked. These organic compounds are crucial for various biochemical processes, such as immune function, energy production, and cell repair. Vitamins help with blood flow, nerve function, and hormone regulation. They boost libido, improve sexual performance, and support overall health. Here's how some vitamins can enhance your passion and vitality.

B Complex: The Energy Ensemble

The B Complex vitamins work together to support sexual health. They increase energy, reduce stress, and improve circulation—all vital for a satisfying sex life. These vitamins are found in whole grains, legumes, nuts, seeds, dark leafy greens, meat, fish, poultry, eggs, and dairy products. Here's the breakdown of the B complex vitamins:

- B1 (Thiamine) improves mood and energy.

- B3 (Niacin) boosts blood flow and lowers cholesterol.

- B6 (Pyridoxine) regulates hormone levels.

- B9 (Folate) supports cell production.

- B12 (Cobalamin) is essential for overall health.

Vitamin C: The Intimacy Enhancer

Vitamin C enhances immune function, helping you stay healthy and energetic. It improves blood flow by strengthening blood vessels and combats oxidative stress, which can affect sexual function. Additionally, Vitamin C supports collagen production, keeping your skin healthy and boosting your confidence. Sources of Vitamin C include citrus fruits (like oranges and lemons), berries (such as strawberries and blueberries), bell peppers, broccoli, and kiwi.

Vitamin D: The Radiance of Love

Vitamin D, known as the "sunshine vitamin," is essential for hormone production, including testosterone and estrogen. Maintaining a healthy hormone balance is vital for a strong libido and optimal sexual function. Vitamin D also supports immune function and bone health. Sources of this vitamin include fatty fish (like salmon and mackerel), egg yolks, fortified dairy products, and sun exposure.

Minerals for Stamina

Minerals may not steal the spotlight, but they're essential for keeping your body in peak condition. These often-overlooked nutrients serve as the building blocks for various bodily functions that directly impact your energy levels, hormonal balance, and overall well-being. Let's take a closer look at five critical minerals that are essential for supporting sexual health and function—zinc, calcium, magnesium, iron, and potassium.

Zinc: The Libido Lifesaver

Zinc is crucial for producing testosterone, a hormone that influences libido in both men and women. Adequate zinc levels help maintain sperm production and mobility in men, improving fertility. In women, zinc supports reproductive health and hormone balance. You can get zinc from oysters, beef, pork, chickpeas, pumpkin seeds, cashews, fortified cereals, and dairy products.

Calcium: The Passion Powerhouse

Calcium is essential for nerve function and muscle contractions, both of which play a critical role in sexual arousal and performance. Adequate calcium levels help regulate the release of neurotransmitters that facilitate communication between the brain and reproductive organs, enhancing sexual responsiveness. Additionally, calcium supports overall cardiovascular health, ensuring proper blood flow, which is vital for maintaining sexual function. Calcium is found in dairy products (like milk, cheese, and yogurt), leafy greens (such as kale and spinach), almonds, and fortified plant-based milk.

Magnesium: The Intimacy Relaxer

Magnesium helps relax muscles and blood vessels, improve circulation, and reduce stress—factors necessary for a satisfying sexual experience. It also supports energy production and hormone balance, giving you the stamina and desire for intimacy. Magnesium sources include dark chocolate, avocados, nuts (like almonds and cashews), whole grains (such as brown rice and quinoa), and legumes (like black beans and chickpeas).

Iron: The Vitality Booster

Iron is needed to produce hemoglobin, the protein in red blood cells that carries oxygen throughout your body. Adequate iron levels ensure your tissues, including those involved in sexual activity, are well-oxygenated and energized. Iron deficiency can lead to fatigue and reduced libido, so it's crucial to maintain sufficient iron levels for sexual health. Iron is found in red meat, poultry, fish, lentils, beans, fortified cereals, spinach, and other leafy greens.

Potassium: The Heart and Muscle Regulator

Potassium is crucial for maintaining healthy blood pressure and proper circulation, both of which are essential for optimal sexual function. It helps regulate muscle contractions, including those involved in sexual activity, and ensures nerve signals are transmitted efficiently. Adequate potassium levels also support overall energy levels, reducing fatigue and enhancing stamina, positively impacting sexual performance and endurance. Potassium-rich foods include bananas, potatoes, spinach, avocados, oranges, and yogurt.

Tips:

- **Fill Your Plate with Fruits and Vegetables:** Make fruits and vegetables the foundation of your meals, as these nutrient-rich foods are packed with antioxidants, vitamins, and minerals that boost sexual function and vitality. Aim to eat a colorful variety to ensure you get a broad spectrum of nutrients that can enhance libido, energy levels, and overall health.

- **Choose Lean Proteins and Healthy Fats:** Select lean proteins, such as chicken, fish, or plant-based sources, and pair them with healthy fats like avocado, olive oil, and nuts. Protein supports muscle health and energy production, both essential for stamina during sexual activity, while healthy fats are key to hormone regulation and promoting a healthy libido. Incorporating lean proteins and healthy fats into your diet will fuel your body for optimal sexual performance.

CHAPTER 7

Aphrodisiac Magic

> *"Aphrodisiacs are like spices; they add flavor, but they aren't the main course."*
>
> — Catherine Zeta-Jones, American Actress

Arousing Energy of Food

For centuries, different cultures have celebrated the erotic power of food. Certain foods and herbs are known for their ability to spark romance and boost libido. Aphrodisiacs are often thought of as magical substances that enhance desire, passion, and sexual performance.

In 1996, the U.S. Food and Drug Administration defined an aphrodisiac as "a food, drink, drug, scent, or device that can arouse or increase sexual desire or libido." Historical figures like Cleopatra indulged in foods like raw oysters and caviar to boost libido. Casanova famously shared oysters with his lovers to spark their sexual interest. Madame Pompadour enjoyed truffles, vanilla, and celery to heighten her desire for Louis XIV. Similarly, Greek and Roman cultures consumed ripe fruits and exotic dishes to enhance their sensual experiences.

The use of food as an aphrodisiac is more than just a myth. Certain foods can influence biological factors like hormone production, blood flow, and energy levels, which are critical for sexual functioning. Additionally, the sensory experience of food—the taste, aroma, and texture—can have a powerful psychological effect, enhancing mood and arousal.

The right foods can elevate desire and improve sexual wellness, making your meals an integral part of your overall sexual health strategy. Incorporating known aphrodisiacs into your diet can boost libido, improve performance, and enhance sexual pleasure. Let's look at some popular aphrodisiacs and their potential sexual health benefits.

Foods That Turn You On!

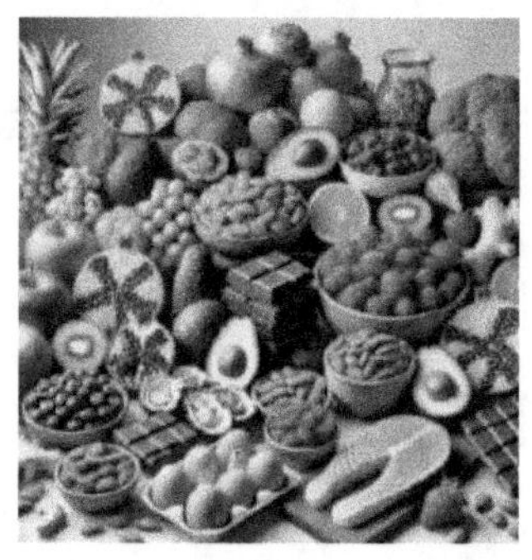

- Dark Chocolate
- Truffles
- Oysters
- Pine Nuts
- Strawberries
- Acai Berries
- Watermelon
- Raspberries
- Pomegranate
- Avocado
- Cherries
- Figs
- Chili Peppers
- Asparagus
- Caviar
- Cinnamon
- Honey
- Ginger
- Maca Root
- Mackerel
- Almonds
- Salmon
- Bananas
- Ginseng
- Basil
- Celery
- Cucumbers
- Beets
- Mint
- Fenugreek
- Saffron
- Garlic
- Vanilla

Oysters: The Ultimate Passion Igniter

Oysters are famously associated with passion and have a long history as an aphrodisiac across various cultures. The legend of oysters as a symbol of love dates back to Greek mythology, where Aphrodite, the goddess of love and beauty, was said to have emerged from the sea on an oyster shell. The word "aphrodisiac" itself comes from Aphrodite's name. The Romans embraced this belief, with the elite often enjoying oysters at feasts and orgies—convinced of their ability to boost sexual performance. During the Renaissance, the notorious Italian lover Casanova was reputed to consume large quantities of oysters daily to maintain his legendary virility.

Oysters are a luxurious delicacy crafted from the unfertilized eggs of female sturgeon and paddlefish, two of the oldest and largest fish species on earth. Their slightly salty-sweet scent is similar to a potent female pheromone, which has been shown to have a sexually stimulating effect. Additionally, the oyster's appearance bears a resemblance to the female genitalia, adding to its erotic allure. Rich in zinc, oysters are crucial in testosterone production and sperm health. They also contain amino acids that trigger the release of sex hormones, further enhancing sexual desire.

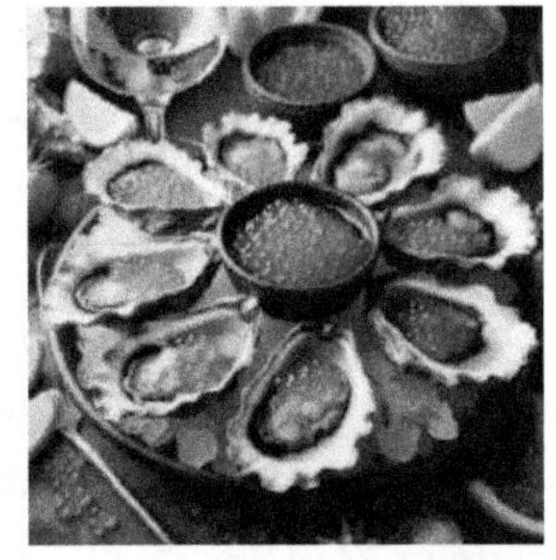

Fun Fact! Oysters change gender multiple times throughout their lives, adding to their mystique and reputation for sexual fluidity and vitality. Enjoying oysters can be a delightful and sensual experience with a partner, enhancing your passion and connection.

Caviar: The Pinnacle of Extravagance

Caviar has been a symbol of luxury and opulence since ancient times, cherished by Persians and Greeks as a delicacy. Throughout history, eggs have been associated with fertility and the potential for life, further elevating caviar's esteemed status. Today, caviar remains a symbol of indulgence and pleasure, enjoyed by royals and aristocrats.

Caviar is rich in protein, iron, zinc, and vitamins A, D, E, B6, and B12. It also contains essential nutrients like magnesium and potassium, which promote overall health and vitality. These nutrients boost libido and enhance sexual health, making caviar a luxurious treat. Indulge in the pairing of caviar and smoked salmon for an elegant appetizer that sets a romantic mood.

Fun Fact! Caviar was once so plentiful in the United States that it was served as a free snack in bars. Its high salt content encouraged patrons to drink more, making it a popular and practical choice for bar owners.

Truffles: The Symbol of Sophistication

Truffles have been prized for their rarity and distinct aroma. The Greeks and Romans considered them a delicacy and an aphrodisiac, using them in feasts to signify luxury and indulgence. In medieval Europe, truffles were associated with nobility and high social status, symbolizing sophistication and romance.

Truffles, renowned for their earthy, musky aroma, have long been celebrated for their aphrodisiac qualities. Their intoxicating scent is believed to mimic pheromones, with androsterone—a hormone found in truffles—thought to stimulate sexual attraction and desire. This luxurious delicacy not only tantalizes the senses but also heightens the mood, making it a prized addition to romantic dining experiences. The allure of truffles lies not only in their unique flavor but in their ability to subtly enhance the chemistry between partners.

Fun Fact! Due to their rarity and high value, truffles are called "black diamonds" in France. They are often hunted with trained dogs or pigs that sniff out these hidden treasures beneath the forest floor—adding an element of adventure and exclusivity to their consumption.

Asparagus: The Timeless Fertility Booster

Asparagus has been celebrated as an aphrodisiac since ancient times. The Greeks and Romans valued its stimulating properties, often serving it at wedding feasts to promote a passionate union. Its reputation for enhancing desire has endured, making asparagus a timeless symbol of love and fertility.

Asparagus has earned its reputation as a natural aphrodisiac, not only because of its suggestive shape but also due to its rich nutritional profile that supports sexual health. Packed with vitamins such as A, C, E, and B6, along with minerals like potassium and folate, asparagus boosts energy levels, enhances circulation, and aids in hormone production—all essential for sexual vitality.

Fun Fact! In the 19th century, French bridegrooms were served three courses of asparagus at their prenuptial dinners. This tradition was believed to boost their libido and ensure a passionate wedding night, highlighting asparagus's long-standing reputation as a potent aphrodisiac.

Watermelon: The Refreshing Arouser

Watermelon has been cultivated for thousands of years, originating in ancient Africa and spreading to the Mediterranean region. In ancient Egypt, it was often placed in tombs as a source of sustenance in the afterlife. Watermelon is celebrated for its refreshing taste, hydrating qualities, and health benefits.

Watermelon is rich in citrulline, an amino acid that boosts blood flow and circulation—similar to the effects of popular erectile dysfunction medications. It also contains vitamins A, B6, and C, supporting overall health and energy levels. Its hydrating properties make watermelon a delicious way to stay in shape and enhance vitality and intimacy. Its refreshing taste and hydrating properties make it a light, energizing addition to any romantic meal.

Fun Fact! In China, watermelon seeds are eaten during the New Year to symbolize fertility and prosperity. The fruit's vibrant red flesh and sweet flavor make it a popular choice for summer celebrations and romantic picnics, enhancing its reputation as a food that can boost love and desire.

Avocados: Nature's Desire Enhancer

Originally cultivated in Central and South America, avocados were named "ahuacatl" by the Aztecs, which means "testicle" due to their shape and esteemed aphrodisiac qualities. The Aztecs valued avocados for their unique appearance and ability to enhance desire and vitality.

Avocados are a nutritional powerhouse. They are rich in healthy fats, vitamin B6, and folic acid, contributing to increased energy and stamina. The potassium in avocados is especially beneficial for boosting libido as it helps regulate blood pressure and improve circulation.

Fun Fact! The Spanish conquistadors were so convinced of avocados' aphrodisiac properties that Catholic priests banned their consumption. This historical belief in avocados' ability to stimulate desire has lasted throughout the ages. Today, avocados are celebrated for their delicious taste, health benefits, and intriguing history as symbols of love and fertility.

Dark Chocolate: The Virility Amplifier

Dark chocolate's reputation as an aphrodisiac dates back to the Aztecs, who saw it as a powerful stimulant. Aztec emperor Montezuma II was known to consume large quantities of cocoa beans to enhance his romantic prowess, believing it boosted his virility and energy.

Dark chocolate is packed with compounds that stimulate mood and sexual desire. It contains phenylethylamine (PEA), a chemical that releases endorphins and mimics the feelings of love. Additionally, the flavonoids in dark chocolate improve blood flow by relaxing blood vessels.

Fun Fact! The scientific name of the cacao tree, Theobroma cacao, means "food of the gods," reflecting its revered status and historical significance across cultures.

Strawberries: The Sweet Symbol of Romance

Strawberries have been celebrated as an edible aphrodisiac since ancient Rome, where they symbolized Venus, the goddess of love, beauty, and fertility. This association with romance has endured through the ages, making strawberries a timeless symbol of desire.

Strawberries are members of the rose family and are unique as they are the only fruit with seeds on the outside rather than the inside. They are rich in vitamin C and antioxidants, which boost blood flow and promote heart health. Strawberries' vibrant red color and juicy texture add to their sensual appeal, making them a delightful and healthy addition to any romantic occasion. Dip fresh strawberries in dark chocolate for a rich, intimate dessert.

Fun Fact! In France, an ancient tradition involved serving newlyweds a cold soup called borage made of strawberries and soured cream to kindle honeymoon fires and encourage romance.

Figs: Nature's Sweet Aphrodisiac

Figs are cherished for their sweet, succulent flavor and impressive health benefits. In ancient Greece, these fruits were revered as sacred and closely linked to love and lavishness. Their unique shape and abundance of seeds have long 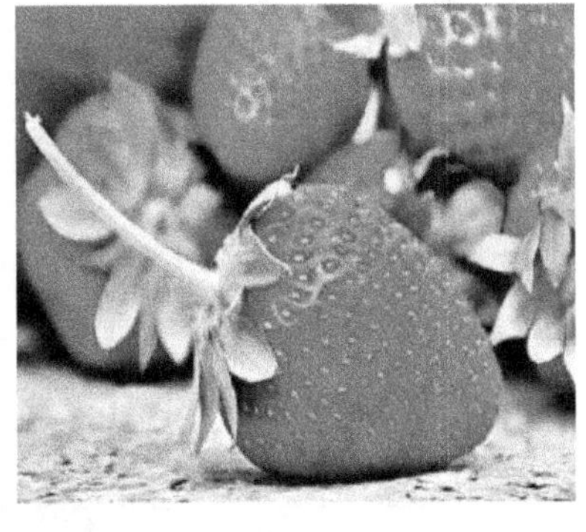 symbolized fertility, making figs a powerful natural aphrodisiac.

Rich in vitamins, minerals, and antioxidants, figs can support reproductive health, improve circulation and blood flow, and enhance sexual vitality. Figs are high in amino acids, which boost libido and improve sexual stamina. They also contain essential vitamins and minerals like magnesium, potassium, and iron, which help maintain energy levels and overall health.

Fun Fact! In ancient times, figs were offered as gifts to gods and used in fertility rituals. The Romans believed figs were a gift from Bacchus, the god of wine and fertility.

Bananas: The Natural Energy Surge

Bananas, with their phallic shape, are often linked to erotic energy across cultures. In Southeast Asia, bananas were among the earliest cultivated fruits.

In the Tantric tradition, bananas symbolize sexual vitality and passion. They are still used in offerings to fertility gods, symbolizing prosperity and fertility.

Bananas contain bromelain, an enzyme that boosts libido and can help reverse impotence in men. They are also rich in potassium and B vitamins, essential for energy production and hormone regulation. These nutrients contribute to vitality and stamina, making bananas a powerful natural aphrodisiac.

Fun Fact! In Central America, the sap of the red banana tree is consumed as an aphrodisiac elixir, believed to enhance sexual desire and performance. This highlights the enduring belief in bananas' ability to ignite passion.

Ginseng: The Ancient Stamina Herb

Ginseng has been valued for thousands of years, especially in traditional Chinese medicine, for its ability to boost energy, improve health, and increase longevity. It gained fame in the Western world in the 17th century for its numerous health benefits.

Ginseng helps the body manage stress, boost energy levels, reduce fatigue, and improve physical performance. It also supports brain function, enhances memory and mental clarity, and strengthens the immune system. As a natural aphrodisiac, ginseng can enhance sexual performance and reduce stress, making it a valuable ally for your romantic life.

Fun Fact! Ginseng roots are known for their distinct shape, often resembling the human body with "arms" and "legs." Ginseng's shape led to the ancient belief that it could heal and restore the entire body. This resemblance and its long history of medicinal use contributed to its reputation as a powerful tonic for overall health and sexual well-being.

Saffron: The Luxurious Spice for Arousal

Saffron, derived from the crocus flower, has been prized for over 3,000 years. Originating in Greece and spreading to Persia, India, and beyond, saffron has been valued for its vibrant color, distinct flavor, and medicinal properties. Ancient civilizations used it for its aphrodisiac qualities. At one time, it was considered more valuable than gold.

Historically, saffron has been used in traditional medicine systems like Ayurveda and Persian medicine to boost libido and treat sexual dysfunction. Due to its potent antioxidant and anti-inflammatory properties, saffron can enhance mood, reduce symptoms of depression, enhance blood flow, balance hormone levels, and improve overall health. Saffron has many potent aphrodisiac qualities, making it a natural enhancer of sexual desire and performance.

Fun Fact! Saffron is one of the most expensive spices in the world, requiring about 75,000 crocus flowers to produce just one pound. It has been used as a perfume, dye, and medicine to treat various ailments, further adding to its luxurious status and unique health benefits.

Maca Root: The Organic Vitality Revitalizer

Maca root, or Peruvian ginseng, has been cherished for over 2,000 years. Originating in the Andes mountains of Peru, it was used by Ancient Incan warriors to boost their strength and stamina before battles.

Maca root is renowned for boosting energy levels, stamina, and endurance. It supports hormonal balance, which can improve mood and reduce menopause symptoms. Additionally, maca enhances sexual function and libido, making it a potent natural aphrodisiac. You can easily add maca to your diet by incorporating it into smoothies, oatmeal, and other foods.

Fun Fact! Maca root comes in various colors, including yellow, red, and black—each offering different health benefits. Often called "Peruvian Viagra," maca is celebrated for its effects on sexual health and libido, gaining worldwide fame as a natural vitality booster.

Garlic: The Endurance Enhancer

Garlic has been valued for its medicinal properties for thousands of years. Ancient civilizations, including the Egyptians, Greeks, and Romans, recognized garlic's health benefits and aphrodisiac qualities. The Egyptians used garlic to boost strength and endurance, the Greeks used it as a remedy for various ailments, and the Romans appreciated its culinary and health-promoting properties.

Garlic is rich in allicin, a compound that improves blood flow and circulation— which enhances sexual performance. It also supports the immune system, helping to fend off illnesses and infections. Its anti-inflammatory and antioxidant properties further boost overall health and vitality.

Fun Fact! Legend states that Tibetan monks were forbidden from entering monasteries if they had eaten garlic. The reason? Garlic was believed to arouse sexual desire, making it incompatible with the monks' vows of celibacy. This underscores the firm belief in garlic's stimulating properties, which has persisted across cultures and centuries.

Basil: The Herb of Love

Basil has long been revered as one of the earth's most noble and sacred plants. The Greeks regarded it as their royal herb, and many professional chefs today still consider it the "king of herbs." In Roman times, basil was more than just an herb—it was a potent

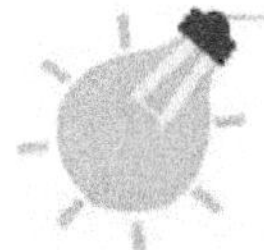

Foods high in antioxidants can combat the effects of aging, improving skin health and vitality

symbol of love and romance. This tradition endures in parts of Italy, where basil is still cherished as a token of affection.

The sweet, aromatic basil leaves were believed to have mystical properties capable of igniting passion and affection. Basil contains high levels of eugenol, which has anti-inflammatory properties, and linalool, which can reduce stress. Its fragrant aroma is believed to be calming, potentially enhancing mood and desire. These qualities make basil a powerful and aromatic addition to romantic occasions.

Fun Fact! In Italy, basil is traditionally a symbol of love. Men would court women by placing a sprig of basil in their hair, signifying their romantic interest and the hope for reciprocation. This charming custom emphasizes basil's enduring association with love and romance.

Honey: Nature's Sexual Health Remedy

Honey has been cherished for centuries, dating back to the Egyptians, Greeks, and Romans. It was often used in religious ceremonies, medicinal practices, and as a natural sweetener. Ancient Egyptians even placed honey in tombs as offerings to the gods for the afterlife.

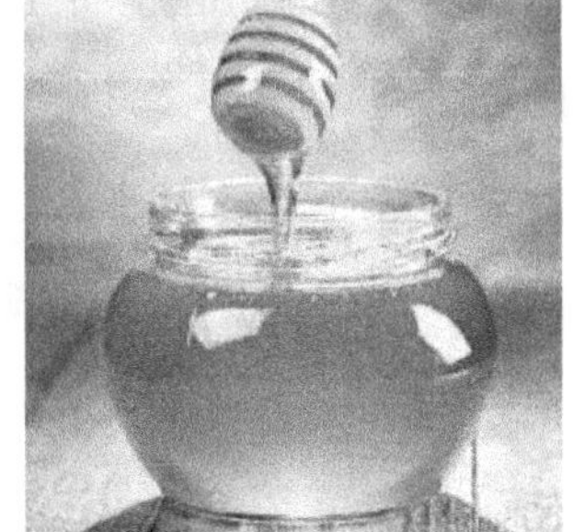

Honey is packed with vitamins, minerals, and antioxidants that promote overall health. Its natural antibacterial and anti-inflammatory properties help heal wounds and soothe sore throats. Honey can also boost energy levels and enhance stamina, making it a natural aphrodisiac. Its natural sugars provide a quick energy boost, while its rich, sweet flavor can add a touch of indulgence to various foods and beverages.

Fun Fact! Archaeologists have found honey pots in ancient Egyptian tombs that are over 3,000 years old and still perfectly edible. This remarkable longevity is due to honey's low moisture content and acidic pH, which create an inhospitable environment for bacteria. Honey's enduring nature and health benefits make it a fascinating and valuable natural aphrodisiac.

Red Wine: The Intimacy Elixir

Red wine has been enjoyed for thousands of years, with its origins tracing back to ancient civilizations like the Egyptians, Greeks, and Romans. It has long been associated with celebrations, rituals, and medicinal purposes.

Red wine is rich in antioxidants, particularly resveratrol, found in the skin of red grapes. These antioxidants help protect your heart by reducing inflammation and preventing damage to blood vessels. In moderation, red wine can also improve blood flow and relax the body, creating the perfect atmosphere for intimacy.

Fun Fact! The famous seducer Casanova reportedly used red wine as part of his romantic endeavors! He believed it enhanced passion and pleasure, proving that red wine's aphrodisiac reputation has long been a part of seductive lore.

Case History: Cindy and Bob's Sweet Journey

Among the lively residents of The Villages, I met Cindy and Bob, a delightful older Italian couple from Ohio. They stood out for their lively dinner parties filled with great company, laughter, delicious dishes, and plenty of homemade wine. One evening, Bob started feeling poorly. "I thought it was just my love for desserts catching up with me," he teased. A check-up with the doctor revealed Bob had diabetes.

The diagnosis was shocking, but Cindy and Bob faced it with their trademark humor and resilience. "Looks like we'll be swapping our wine for water and cake for kale," Cindy said with a laugh. Bob, ever the jokester, added, "I guess my sweet tooth finally bit back!"

Managing diabetes required a major overhaul of their diet and lifestyle. They took nutrition classes together and learned about carbohydrates, the glycemic index, and balanced meals. "Who knew we'd become experts on quinoa and chia seeds in our 60s?" Bob quipped. They carefully planned their meals to ensure Bob received the proper nutrients without spiking his blood sugar.

Cindy was incredibly supportive, adapting their favorite recipes to be diabetes-friendly. "I never thought I'd say this, but I've started to enjoy kale," she joked. They transformed their kitchen into a testing ground for new dishes and flavors. "Our date nights now involve cooking competitions—healthy style," Bob laughed.

Diabetes introduced challenges that extended far beyond dietary adjustments, deeply affecting Bob's sexual health. "It's hard to feel sexy when you're worried about your blood sugar," he admitted. They sought advice from their doctor, who emphasized the importance of communication. "Communication is key," Cindy said, "and sometimes a little humor goes a long way."

Despite the challenges, their relationship remained strong. "We might have to plan a bit more, but our love life is as vibrant as ever," Cindy winked. They focused on maintaining their emotional and physical connection, rediscovering the art of kissing. "It's amazing how something so simple can be so powerful," Bob grinned.

Key Lessons:

- **Face Challenges with Humor and Positivity:** Bob and Cindy approached his diabetes diagnosis with resilience and a sense of humor, helping them face the difficulties together. Their light-hearted attitude shows the value of staying positive during tough times.

- **Adapt and Support One Another:** Bob and Cindy adapted their lifestyle by learning about diabetes, trying new recipes, and supporting each other through dietary changes. This emphasizes the importance of mutual support and adaptability in managing health challenges.

- **Prioritize Communication and Intimacy:** Despite the impact of diabetes on their sexual health, Bob and Cindy maintained open communication and worked to preserve their intimate connection. Their approach highlights the need for honest discussions and creative solutions to sustain closeness in relationships.

Eat Smart in The Villages

In The Villages, where energy and vitality reign supreme, eating well is more than just maintaining health—it's about nurturing your body for a vibrant life. A balanced diet rich in nutrients supports overall well-being—helping maintain a healthy weight, boost immune function, and elevate mood.

Cooking at home is the cornerstone of a healthy lifestyle, offering unparalleled control over what goes into your meals. By preparing your own food, you can carefully choose fresh, wholesome ingredients, manage portion sizes, and steer clear of hidden sugars, unhealthy fats, and unnecessary additives often found in restaurants or pre-packaged meals. Plus, home cooking ensures a well-rounded intake of essential vitamins and minerals that support your overall well-being.

Beyond its nutritional benefits, cooking can be an enjoyable and therapeutic activity. It offers the chance to experiment with new, healthy recipes, explore exciting flavors, and tap into your creativity in the kitchen. This mindful approach to cooking enhances your physical health and boosts mental well-being, fostering a sense of accomplishment and joy. By embracing home cooking, you're nurturing your body and mind, setting the stage for a more vibrant, energized life.

In The Villages, men and women have different cooking habits. For the women, 67% whip up homemade meals daily, 26% cook at least once a week, and only 7% cook just once a month or less.
Men take a different approach to their eating habits. About 47% cook daily, 32% cook weekly, and 16% make meals at home just once a month or not at all—often choosing to eat out instead.

Tips:

- **Spice Up Your Diet with Aphrodisiacs**: Elevate your meals by incorporating natural aphrodisiac foods like dark chocolate, oysters, and strawberries. These delicious treats not only tantalize the taste buds but also help stimulate the senses and boost blood flow, enhancing arousal and intimacy.

- **Harness the Power of Nutrient-Rich Foods**: Fuel your sexual vitality with nutrient-dense foods like almonds, avocados, and garlic—rich in zinc, vitamin E, and healthy fats. These foods work synergistically to balance hormones, increase energy levels, and improve overall sexual function, ensuring enhanced performance and greater satisfaction in the bedroom.

CHAPTER 8

Sexercise

"Sex is like exercise; it's good for you."
— Jack LaLanne, American Health Expert

Sweating for Pleasure

Exercise isn't just for staying fit—it's a game-changer for your sex life! Regular physical activity elevates stamina, energy levels, and overall vitality, making intimate moments more exciting and enjoyable. When you work out, your body releases endorphins—nature's feel-good hormones—that enhance pleasure, reduce stress, and even increase sexual desire. Since sexual activity engages your entire body, keeping muscles toned, blood flowing efficiently, and nerves functioning optimally through exercise is essential for peak performance.

Cardiovascular exercises like running, swimming, or cycling significantly improve circulation, ensuring blood flows to all the right places to enhance arousal and sexual performance. Strength training helps build muscle tone, power, and endurance, providing you with better physical control and stamina during intimacy. Flexibility, stretching, and balance exercises, like yoga and Pilates, improve agility and range of motion, allowing you to explore different positions more comfortably and confidently. Incorporating pelvic floor exercises, such as Kegels, strengthens the muscles that play a crucial role in sexual function, leading to increased control, endurance, and heightened sensations during intimacy.

Beyond the benefits of physical health, regular exercise also supports mental well-being. Regular workouts can reduce anxiety, elevate mood, and build self-confidence, all of which contribute to a more fulfilling and satisfying sex life.

Incorporating a mix of cardiovascular, strength training, flexibility, stretching, balance work, and pelvic floor exercises into your routine can boost your fitness and improve your sexual health and enjoyment.

Get Your Heart Pumping

Aerobic exercise goes beyond just getting your heart pumping; it's about refreshing your body, filling you with energy, and boosting your vitality. Known as cardiovascular or endurance training, this type of workout is the cornerstone of any well-rounded fitness plan. Think of it as the ultimate tune-up for your

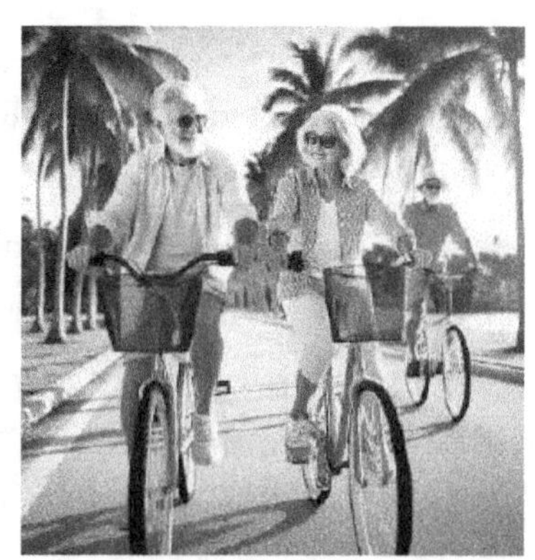

engine, keeping everything running smoothly and efficiently. Aerobic exercise offers numerous benefits, from boosting your mood and energy levels to improving cardiovascular health and increasing lung capacity.

Whether dancing, running, cycling, or swimming, each purposeful movement helps you shake off stress, strengthen your heart, and build endurance. Aerobic exercise revitalizes your body and mind, making you feel more alive with every step, pedal, or stroke. So, lace up your sneakers, dive into the pool, or hit the pavement—let aerobic exercise energize and transform you from the inside out.

How to Perform Aerobic Activities:

Walking and Jogging

- Start with a brisk walk or light jog in a comfortable environment, like a park or on a treadmill.

- Gradually increase your pace to elevate your heart rate and improve cardiovascular health.

- Aim for 20-30 minutes of walking or jogging at least three to five days a week for optimal results.

Swimming

- Dive into a pool for lap swimming or join a water aerobics class to enjoy a low-impact, full-body workout.

- Swimming is gentle on the joints while providing excellent cardiovascular and muscle-toning benefits.

- Swim for 20-30 minutes, two to three times a week, to boost endurance and overall fitness.

Cycling

- Jump on a stationary bike or ride your bicycle outdoors for a fun, effective workout.

- Start at a moderate pace and adjust the resistance or incline as you build strength.

- Cycle for 30-45 minutes, three to five times a week, to improve stamina and leg strength.

Dancing

- Join a dance class or groove to your favorite tunes at home.

- Styles like salsa, Zumba, and ballroom dancing offer both aerobic exercise and fun social interaction.

- Dance for at least 20-30 minutes weekly to boost your heart rate and enhance flexibility and coordination.

Pump It Up

Strength training isn't just about pumping iron—it's a transformative journey for your body and sexual vitality. Known as resistance or weight-bearing training, this type of workout is essential to a comprehensive fitness plan.

Strength training sculpts and tones muscles, enhancing your physical appearance and self-assurance. These are vital ingredients for sexual attraction and desire, creating a positive boost of confidence that can significantly enhance your intimate relationships. Building strength and improving your physique will allow you to look better and feel more confident, making you more attractive and desirable.

Building muscle strength also means greater stamina and endurance, which are crucial for those marathon moments of intimacy. Like aerobic exercise, strength training increases blood flow, ensuring essential oxygen and nutrients reach every body part—including those vital for arousal and sexual performance.

Strength training is essential for supporting hormone balance. It helps increase testosterone levels, which plays a key role in maintaining a healthy libido and optimal sexual function for both men and women. Proper hormone balance is crucial for sustaining a strong sex drive.

Exercises like push-ups, pull-ups, and planks also strengthen the core, improving posture and stability. Better posture enhances your appearance, and increased strength can boost self-confidence. This added confidence can positively impact your overall sexual appeal.

Including strength training in your routine two to three times a week creates a well-rounded fitness plan. Beyond building muscle, these exercises can elevate your confidence and sexual vitality, making it a valuable addition to your fitness and intimate life.

How to Perform Strength Training:

Weightlifting (Squats, Deadlifts, Bench Presses, Bicep Curls)

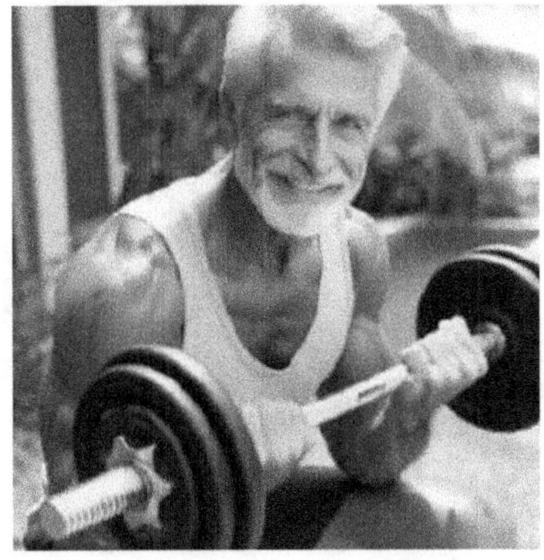

- Begin with a weight that challenges your muscles but still allows you to maintain proper form throughout each movement.

- Aim for 8-12 repetitions per exercise, completing 2-3 sets for optimal muscle engagement and growth.

- Focus on maintaining correct posture and breathing techniques to maximize results and prevent injury. Exhale during exertion and inhale on the return phase of each lift.

Resistance Band Exercises

- Secure the resistance band under your feet or around a stable object to create tension.

- Target all major muscle groups—legs, back, chest, arms, shoulders, and core—by pulling the band upwards or outwards, depending on the exercise.

- Perform 10-15 repetitions for each movement, adjusting the resistance band's tension to ensure it provides a suitable challenge. Increase resistance as your strength improves for continued progress.

Body-Weight Exercises (Push-ups, Pull-ups, Planks, Lunges)

- Begin with the foundational form for each exercise, paying close attention to proper alignment and muscle engagement to prevent injury and ensure effectiveness.

- As you build strength, gradually increase the number of repetitions or incorporate variations like incline push-ups, walking lunges, or side planks for a greater challenge.

- Aim for 10-15 repetitions per set, completing 2-3 sets per exercise for balanced muscle development and endurance.

Kettlebell Training

- Select a kettlebell weight that matches your fitness level while still providing a challenge.

- Incorporate exercises such as kettlebell swings, goblet squats, or Turkish get-ups, ensuring controlled movements to fully engage your muscles.

- Prioritize proper technique and range of motion to reduce the risk of injury and gain the most from each exercise. As you progress, gradually increase the weight or intensity to continue building strength and endurance.

Flex Your Way to Fun

Flexibility exercises are a key part of any well-rounded fitness routine, offering benefits that extend far beyond physical fitness. By increasing range of motion and loosening tight muscles, these exercises improve posture and mobility and reduce the risk of injury. Flexibility training also plays an important role in enhancing sexual health, as it promotes greater ease and comfort during intimate moments by reducing tension in areas like the hips, lower back, and pelvis.

Making flexibility a priority can help boost joint mobility and muscle pliability, making everyday movements smoother and less painful. Regular stretching improves comfort in daily activities and strengthens muscles and connective tissues, reducing the likelihood of strains and injuries.

For those dealing with chronic pain, such as lower back discomfort, daily flexibility exercises can be particularly helpful. These exercises improve posture and reduce the risk of recurring pain by easing muscle tension and improving body alignment.

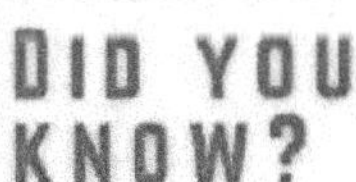
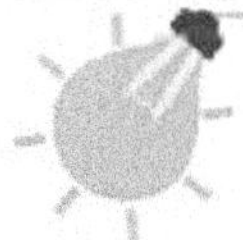

In addition to physical benefits, flexibility exercises, like yoga and stretching, are powerful tools for reducing stress and anxiety. Reducing stress can help alleviate performance pressure, making it easier to enjoy intimate moments with greater comfort and confidence. This creates an environment that enhances sexual desire and satisfaction.

How to Perform Flexibility Exercises:

Static Stretching (Hamstring, Calf, Shoulder)

Static stretching involves holding a position that gently elongates the muscles, promoting flexibility and relaxation.

- Hold each stretch for 15-30 seconds, concentrating on fully lengthening the muscle.

- Focus on deep, controlled breathing to help your muscles relax. Avoid bouncing or jerking movements to prevent injury.

- Repeat each stretch 2-3 times, gently increasing the stretch as your muscles loosen up. This type of stretching is ideal for improving flexibility and can be performed after a workout or as part of a daily routine.

Dynamic Stretching (Leg Swings, Arm Circles, Torso Twists)

Dynamic stretching involves moving your body through a full range of motion, preparing muscles and joints for more intense activity.

- Move your limbs through a controlled range of motion, starting with smaller movements.

- Gradually increase the reach or speed of the movements as your muscles warm up.

- Perform dynamic stretches for 5-10 minutes, either before exercise to warm up or after to aid in recovery. This type of stretching is great for enhancing mobility and preparing the body for physical activity.

Balance for Bedroom Bliss

Balance exercises focus on improving your body's ability to maintain stability and coordination. Incorporating them into your routine enhances your strength and posture, supporting everyday movements and promoting better control and flexibility. These benefits improve your overall health by reducing the risk of falls and injuries, while also enhancing your sexual health by boosting confidence, stamina, and body awareness. Balance exercises are a simple way to support a healthier, more active lifestyle, helping you feel more connected and comfortable in your daily activities and intimate moments.

How to Perform Balance Exercises:

Standing on One Leg

- Begin by standing tall with your feet hip-width apart and your weight evenly distributed.

- Slowly lift one foot off the ground, balancing on the opposite leg.

- Hold this position for 30 seconds, keeping your core engaged and your gaze forward. Then, switch to the other leg.

- As you build strength and balance, challenge yourself by gradually increasing the time you can hold the position or by closing your eyes for added difficulty.

Heel-to-Toe Walk (Tandem Walking)

- Stand upright with one foot placed directly in front of the other, so your heel touches the toes of the back foot.

- Keep your arms by your sides or on your hips for balance.

- Take slow, controlled steps, ensuring the heel of your front foot touches the toes of your back foot with each step.

- Aim for 10-20 steps in a straight line, focusing on maintaining balance and coordination throughout the exercise.

- This exercise is excellent for improving stability and coordination, making it useful for daily movements and overall agility.

Side Leg Raises

- Stand tall next to a sturdy chair or wall for balance support. Slowly lift one leg out to the side, keeping it straight and your toes pointing forward.

- Focus on controlled movement, engaging your core and hip muscles.

- Hold the lifted position for a moment before gently lowering your leg back down.

- Repeat on the opposite side, aiming for 10-15 repetitions on each leg.

- This exercise strengthens the muscles around the hips, improves balance, and enhances stability, making it a great addition to any routine.

Tai Chi (Slow, Controlled Movements)

- Find a quiet, open space where you can move freely without distractions or obstacles.

- Begin with the basic Tai Chi stance: stand with your feet shoulder-width apart, knees slightly bent, and arms relaxed by your sides.

- Follow a Tai Chi routine or series of movements, concentrating on slow, graceful, and deliberate motions.

- Focus on your breathing and body alignment, allowing each movement to flow seamlessly into the next.

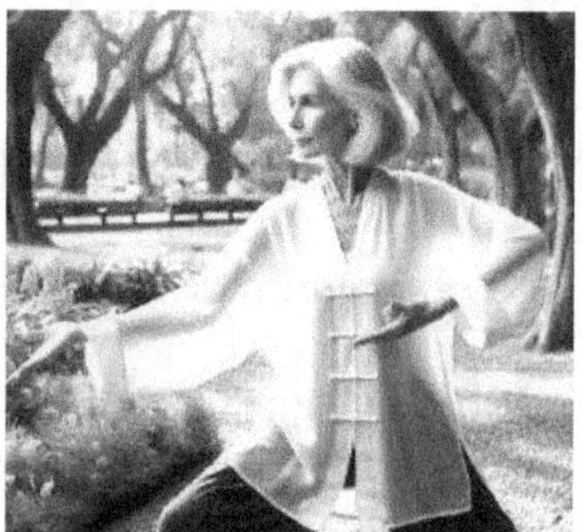

- Tai Chi promotes balance, coordination, and relaxation while improving body awareness and mental clarity.

- Practice for 15-30 minutes to fully experience its calming and health-enhancing benefits.

Mastering Kegels

Have you heard about Kegels? If not, prepare to be amazed by how these simple yet powerful exercises can transform your well-being! Kegels target the pelvic floor muscles, which are vital in supporting bladder control, core strength, and sexual function. If you've ever experienced an unexpected leak when you coughed or sneezed, you're not alone—this common issue, known as stress incontinence, affects many people as they age due to weakened pelvic muscles. Regularly practicing Kegels strengthens these muscles, reducing incontinence, enhancing overall core stability, and promoting better circulation. Not only do Kegels help with bladder control, but they also improve sexual health by increasing sensitivity, boosting arousal, and even contributing to more satisfying orgasms.

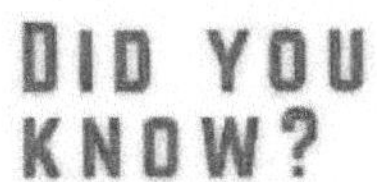
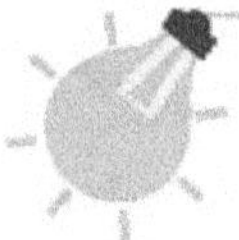

How to Perform Kegel Exercises:

1. **Locate Your Pelvic Floor Muscles**

   o To identify your pelvic floor muscles, try stopping the flow of urine midstream during urination. The muscles you engage to do this are your pelvic floor muscles.

2. **Prepare for Exercise**

    o   Ensure your bladder is empty, then find a comfortable position, either seated or lying down, where you can focus on the exercise without distractions.

3. **Perform the Exercise**

    o   Contract your pelvic floor muscles by squeezing them as if you were lifting them upward and inward.

    o   Hold the contraction for 3-5 seconds, keeping the effort controlled and steady.

4. **Maintain Proper Technique**

    o   Focus solely on engaging your pelvic floor muscles without tightening your abdomen, thighs, or buttocks.

    o   Maintain a natural breathing pattern and avoid holding your breath during the exercise.

5. **Build Consistency**

    o   Incorporate Kegel exercises into your daily routine. Aim for three sets each day for the best results.

    o   Be patient and persistent, as noticeable improvements in bladder control or sexual function may take a few weeks of regular practice.

Case History: Ginger's Road to Health

In The Villages I had the pleasure of meeting Marilyn, known to her friends as "Ginger," during happy hour one evening at Spanish Springs Town Square—a free-spirited soul who never married and embraced life with gusto. Ginger was always the life of the party, effortlessly dancing and chatting at every social gathering. During one of these lively happy hour meetups, Ginger pulled me aside with a little confession. She had just received some unexpected news—high blood pressure. "Looks like my body isn't as indestructible as my spirit," she joked, her playful attitude still intact. "Guess it's time to hit the gym."

True to her nature, Ginger took on this challenge with humor and determination. "If I'm doing this, I'm going all in," she declared. And she wasn't kidding. From aerobics to weight training, Ginger threw herself into her new fitness routine, quickly becoming a regular at various classes. "I haven't moved this much since the disco days!" she laughed. Weightlifting, however, was a whole new experience for her. "Lifting weights is like lifting my mood," she quipped, flexing her biceps with a grin.

Ginger's real game changer came with strength training and Kegel exercises. "Who knew you could work out and spice up your love life at the same time?" she teased, her mischievous smile saying it all. As she learned more about the benefits of Kegels, Ginger discovered that strengthening her pelvic floor did more than improve her bladder control—it revitalized her sexual health. "It's like getting a two-for-one deal at the gym," she winked. Ginger was thrilled by how exercise boosted her strength and put the spark back in her intimate life.

Ginger started encouraging her friends to embrace the same journey. "Exercise has put the spring back in my step and the spark back in the bedroom!" she confided. She advocated for healthy living, using humor to get her peers talking about topics often brushed aside, like sexual health.

Despite the initial challenges, Ginger found joy in her new routine. "I never thought I'd say this, but I actually love working out now!" she admitted. Soon, her zest for life was spreading throughout the community. "I'm living proof it's never too late to take care of yourself," she proclaimed proudly. Ginger's journey reminds us that health and happiness are always within reach, regardless of age.

Key Lessons:

- **Stay Positive and Resilient**: Ginger faced her health challenges with humor and a strong spirit. Her ability to find laughter during difficult times shows how a positive mindset can make even the toughest situations easier.

- **Commit to Wellness**: Ginger prioritized her health, following a routine of aerobic exercise, strength training, and Kegels. This dedication significantly improved her overall well-being and energy.

- **Promote Open Conversations**: Ginger was a firm believer in openly discussing her blood pressure issues and how they affected her sexual health. She encouraged others to speak up about similar topics, breaking the silence around intimate health concerns. She empowered others to face their own challenges with confidence and take control of their well-being.

Sneak in More Movement

Maintaining your vitality as you age isn't about luck—it's about making physical activity a regular part of your life. The good news is that there are plenty of options, each offering benefits that go beyond just staying fit. By committing to an active lifestyle, you improve not only your physical health but your overall sense of well-being.

Start with simple activities like walking or swimming to get your heart pumping and increase your stamina. Add strength training to build muscle and protect your bones from weakening as you age. Stretching is equally important, as it helps maintain flexibility and ensures ease of movement in your daily tasks.

And don't forget Kegel exercises! These easy, discreet exercises strengthen your pelvic floor, improving bladder control and supporting sexual health. You can do them anytime—while brushing your teeth or watching TV. The key to success is consistency, so set reminders, stay dedicated, and celebrate the improvements you notice along the way!

Exercise doesn't have to mean hitting the gym. You can incorporate movement into your daily routine—take the stairs instead of the elevator, park farther from your destination, or turn conversations into walking chats. Even your hobbies can keep you active—golf swings, tennis matches, or gardening all count. The key is to keep your body moving, lift your mood, and support your heart health.

The best part is that exercise isn't one-size-fits-all. Listen to your body, start at your own pace, and gradually increase the intensity as you become more fit. Remember, staying active is a powerful step toward better sexual health and overall well-being. The journey begins with your commitment to making physical activity a natural part of your lifestyle.

Tips:

- **Boost Your Sexual Health with Aerobic Exercise**: Regular aerobic activities like walking, swimming, or cycling increase blood flow, enhance stamina, and boost energy—all of which can improve sexual performance and endurance.

- **Strengthen Your Body with Anaerobic Exercise**: Add anaerobic exercises and Kegels to your routine to build strength, improve flexibility, and maintain a strong pelvic floor, supporting better sexual function and overall health.

CHAPTER 9

Mood Swings and Mattress Springs

*"When it comes to sex, the most important six inches
are the ones between the ears."*

— Dr. Ruth Westheimer, German-American Sex Therapist

Mind Over Desire

Embark on a vibrant journey through life where your mental health profoundly shapes your sexual experiences as you age. In The Villages, the quality of your intimate relationships and social connections plays a pivotal role in your sex life. Relationships grounded in respect, open communication, and emotional intimacy often lead to greater sexual activity and satisfaction. Cherishing and nurturing these connections can significantly enhance happiness and overall life satisfaction. Let's explore how to cultivate these bonds, ensuring your mental well-being and sexual health flourish together for a more fulfilling and joyful life.

Taking care of your mental health is crucial for maintaining a fulfilling sex life. Challenges like depression, anxiety, and loneliness can significantly impact your sexual desire and satisfaction. Depression can feel like a rain cloud, dampening your libido and causing frustration in the bedroom. Anxiety is a persistent critic, whispering doubts about your performance and appearance. Loneliness, often common in older age, can dim the spark of interest in sexual intimacy. These factors highlight the need for holistic care that addresses physical vitality and emotional well-being.

Strained relationships—whether due to conflicts, illness, or loss—can hinder your sexual fulfillment and make it difficult to have open conversations about sexual concerns. The landscape of intimacy is also shaped by dynamics like divorce and remarriage, adding complexity to relationships and expectations around intimacy. Understanding these dynamics is essential for creating a supportive environment where you can openly discuss and address your emotional health needs.

Mental health in The Villages is strong, especially among women. Of the women surveyed, 28% reported having fair to good mental health, 45% described it as very good, and an impressive 27% rated their mental health as excellent.

Men also demonstrated positive mental health outcomes. Around 17% of men rated their mental health as fair to good, 45% said it was very good, and 38% considered their mental health excellent.

Residents of The Villages who reported better mental health also enjoyed a more active and satisfying sex life. Their secret to happiness? Confidence in themselves and their sexuality, which contributed to a more fulfilling and enjoyable intimate life.

These findings reflect a community with a solid foundation of mental well-being for both men and women, with many residents thriving emotionally.

Love Your Body

Society often emphasizes youthful appearances, but aging shows us that wrinkles are badges of wisdom earned through a lifetime of experiences. Embrace your journey and age like fine wine—each wrinkle tells a story of resilience and growth. Don't compare yourself to grape juice; celebrate and savor the richness of your vintage self!

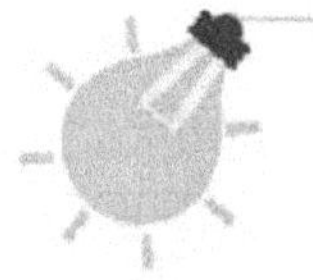

Having a positive body image can improve your sexual experiences and overall satisfaction

As you age, developing a positive body image is crucial. Accepting the changes in your body can significantly improve your self-confidence—particularly in your intimate life. Here are some simple ways to nurture a healthy body image and build sexual self-confidence:

Celebrate Your Body's Journey: Every wrinkle, scar, and mark is a badge of honor, a testament to your life's adventures. These features are not flaws but unique symbols of the experiences and challenges you've conquered, making you beautiful in your own right.

Focus on Strength and Vitality: Rather than fixating on appearance, concentrate on how strong and capable your body is. Engage in activities that make you feel vibrant and energetic, such as walking, biking, or dancing.

Practice Self-Compassion: Treat yourself with the kindness and understanding you would offer a friend. Everyone ages, and changes are a natural part of life. Embracing them with compassion can help you feel more at peace with your body.

Engage in Self-Care: Regular self-care routines can help you feel more in tune with your body and boost your confidence. These include skin and hair care, massages, or simply relaxing and soaking up some Vitamin D.

Confidence in the Sheets

A positive body image boosts sexual confidence and leads to greater satisfaction in intimate relationships. When you feel good about yourself, you can enjoy intimacy more fully. Here's why building your self-confidence is essential:

Better Mental Health: A positive body image lowers stress and anxiety, helping you feel more relaxed and confident in intimate situations.

Stronger Relationships: When you feel good about yourself, you're more open to communicating with your partner, leading to deeper connections and greater comfort during intimate moments.

Increased Libido: Confidence in your body can boost your desire for intimacy, making you more enthusiastic about exploring and enjoying sexual experiences.

In The Villages, men and women have similar views on sexual performance. Over 62% rated their performance as average or below, possibly reflecting modesty or a realistic view of their abilities. On the other hand, 38% of residents—both men and women—felt they were above average in intimacy, showing a strong sense of confidence in this area.

Why does this matter? These insights suggest that while many residents maintain a modest or grounded perspective, many feel empowered and confident. This confidence likely enhances their overall well-being, highlighting how a positive self-image in one area can lead to a greater sense of fulfillment in other aspects of life.

Embracing your aging body with love and respect is a powerful way to boost your sexual self-confidence. Celebrate your unique journey and focus on your strengths. This will allow you to shift your perspective on aging and open the doors to a more fulfilling and intimate life.

Stress Less and Love More

Stress affects more than just your mind—it can also strain your body and relationships. When stress levels rise, it becomes harder to maintain close, intimate connections. Studies show that stress plays a major role in reducing sex drive by disrupting hormone levels. As cortisol increases, it throws off the balance of testosterone and estrogen, leading to a drop in libido and sexual performance.

Mentally, stress brings anxiety and depression, which can further dampen sexual desire and satisfaction. It's like a shadow that makes it hard to enjoy life's brighter moments. Older adults with higher stress levels often report lower sexual desire, difficulty with arousal, and less sexual satisfaction.

The good news is that there are many ways to manage stress. Regular physical activity, relaxation techniques, and open communication can significantly reduce stress levels, boosting your sexual health and overall well-being.

Relax and Recharge

Relaxation practices are powerful tools that help you feel calm and boost your mental health. From deep breathing exercises to guided imagery, these practices lower stress levels and enhance sexual desire. Practicing these techniques regularly can reduce muscle tension and chronic pain, making physical intimacy more comfortable and enjoyable. Relaxation practices also improve concentration and mood, elevating sexual desire and performance. Here are some proven relaxation techniques, along with instructions and their benefits for sexual health:

Deep Breathing Exercises

Deep breathing exercises are simple yet effective methods for calming the mind and body, reducing stress, and promoting relaxation.

How to Practice Deep Breathing:

- Find a Quiet Space: Sit or lie down comfortably in a peaceful environment.

- Close Your Eyes: Minimize external distractions and focus inward.

- Inhale Deeply: Slowly breathe through your nose, fully expanding your lungs and letting your abdomen rise. Count to four as you inhale.

- Hold Your Breath: Hold your breath gently for a count of four.

- Exhale Slowly: Exhale slowly through your mouth, counting to four, and allow your abdomen to fall.

- Repeat: Continue this breathing cycle for 5-10 minutes, focusing on the sensation of each breath.

Benefits of Deep Breathing Exercises

- **Stress Reduction:** When you practice deep breathing, you activate your body's natural relaxation response by engaging the parasympathetic nervous system. This helps calm your mind, reduce stress, and promote well-being. Managing stress is crucial for your sexual health because long-term stress can throw off your body's natural sexual responses. High cortisol levels (the stress hormone) can lower your libido and lead to performance issues.

- **Improved Circulation:** Deep breathing increases oxygen levels in your body and improves circulation, especially to areas like your pelvic region. Good blood flow is key for sexual health, especially as you age. It supports arousal and helps your body respond naturally to sexual stimuli. With better circulation, you can increase sensitivity and boost overall sexual performance, making intimate experiences more pleasurable

- **Enhanced Emotional Connection:** Deep breathing encourages mindfulness, helping you be more present and connected during intimate moments. This mindfulness fosters a deeper emotional bond with your partner, reducing performance anxiety and increasing sexual satisfaction. By being more aware of your body and emotions through deep breathing, you can experience more fulfilling and connected intimate experiences.

Progressive Muscle Relaxation (PMR)

Progressive muscle relaxation (PMR) is another effective technique that involves deliberately tensing and relaxing different muscle groups throughout the body. This method helps alleviate physical tension and reduce overall stress levels.

How to Practice Progressive Muscle Relaxation:

- Find a Comfortable Position: Sit or lie down in a relaxed position.

- Close Your Eyes: Deeply focus on the exercise.

- Tense and Relax Muscle Groups: Start from your toes and work up to your head, tensing each muscle group for about 5 seconds, then slowly release the tension for 10-15 seconds.

- Feet: Curl your toes tightly, then release.

- Calves: Tighten your calf muscles, then release.

- Thighs: Squeeze your thigh muscles, then release.

- Abdomen: Tighten your stomach muscles, then release.

- Hands: Clench your fists, then release.

- Arms: Flex your biceps, then release.

- Shoulders: Raise your shoulders to your ears, then release.

- Face: Tighten your facial muscles (squeeze your eyes shut, clench jaw), then release.

- Focus on Relaxation: Pay attention to the sensation of relaxation as you release each muscle group.

Benefits of Progressive Muscle Relaxation

- **Reduces Tension and Stress:** Focusing on tensing and then relaxing each muscle group with progressive muscle relaxation (PMR) releases physical tension and lowers stress levels. Managing stress is crucial for your sexual health, as high stress can decrease libido and lead to anxiety about intimacy. PMR helps you relax your body and mind, making intimate experiences more comfortable and enjoyable.

- **Improves Body Awareness:** PMR helps you become more aware of your body and the sensations in your muscles. This increased awareness can enhance your ability to tune into your body during intimate moments. For older adults, this can lead to improved sensitivity and a better connection to your sexual responses, making intimacy more satisfying.

- **Boosts Sleep Quality:** PMR promotes deep relaxation, which can also improve your sleep quality. When you're well-rested, energy levels increase and your mood naturally improves. This boost in energy and positive mindset plays a vital role in maintaining a healthy and satisfying sex life. Being well-rested enhances your physical stamina and makes you more emotionally engaged, helping you feel more connected and present during intimate moments. A good night's sleep can make all the difference in keeping your sexual health vibrant and balanced.

Guided Imagery

Guided imagery is a relaxation technique that harnesses the power of the imagination to promote emotional and physical well-being. You can reduce stress, anxiety, and tension by mentally visualizing serene and peaceful environments, such as a quiet beach, a lush forest, or a tranquil mountain lake. This practice encourages the mind to shift focus away from negative or overwhelming thoughts and replace them with calming and peaceful imagery.

How to Practice Guided Imagery:

- Find a Quiet Space: Settle comfortably in a serene environment.

- Close Your Eyes: Focus on the visualization.

- Take Deep Breaths: Begin with a few deep breaths to relax.

- Think of a Peaceful Scene: Visualize a place where you feel calm and happy (a beach, forest, or mountain). Engage all your senses to make the scene vivid.

- Sight: See the colors, light, and objects.

- Sound: Envision the sounds you hear (waves, birds, or wind).

- Smell: Think about scents (saltwater, pine, or flowers).

- Touch: Feel the sensations (a warm sun or a cool breeze).

- Taste: Imagine your favorite flavors (sweet, tangy, or savory).

- Stay in the Scene: Spend several minutes immersed in your scene, allowing yourself to relax deeply.

- Return Slowly: When ready, gently bring your awareness back to the present moment, take a few deep breaths, and open your eyes.

Benefits of Guided Imagery

- **Reduces Stress and Anxiety:** Guided imagery helps you visualize calming and positive scenes, which lowers stress and anxiety levels. Reducing stress is important for your sexual health because high stress can interfere with your desire for intimacy and sexual performance.

- **Improves Focus and Mindfulness:** Guided imagery encourages you to focus on specific mental images, which improves mindfulness and awareness of the present moment. This increased focus can enhance your connection with your partner during intimate times, helping you stay present and engaged. For older adults, this can lead to deeper emotional bonds and more satisfying sexual experiences.

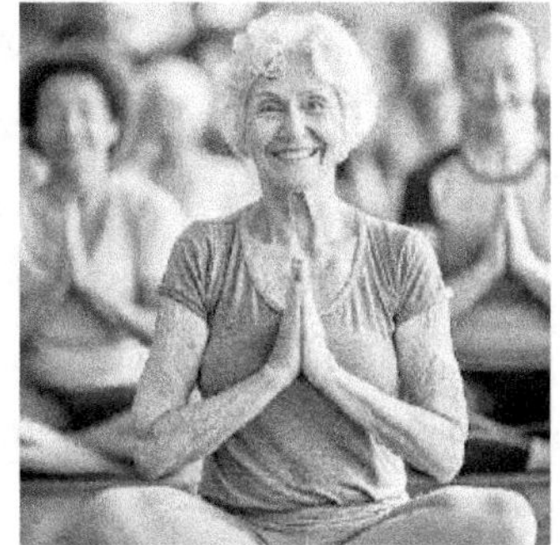

- **Enhances Emotional Well-Being:** Using guided imagery to focus on positive, uplifting thoughts can improve your overall emotional well-being. Feeling emotionally balanced and happy is key to a healthy sex life. When you feel good about yourself and your relationship, you're more likely to experience increased intimacy and sexual satisfaction.

Case History: Mary and Jim's Mindful Voyage

Meet Mary and Jim, a charming and resilient couple from Canada whose love has carried them through life's many challenges. We first met at the Market of Marion, where I found my precious Chihuahua, Martini—she was my first dog and an instant source of joy. Mary and Jim, too, were drawn to the healing power of companionship, adopting a playful Yorkie as their emotional support animal. They shared how their new furry friend would be a comforting presence, helping them navigate their struggles with stress and anxiety.

Mary, a retired nurse, and Jim, a former teacher, found themselves navigating the inevitable challenges that come with aging. The stress and anxiety they experienced began to take a toll on their relationship, pushing them to seek a path toward healing and connection. Determined to overcome these hurdles, they incorporated relaxation techniques into their daily routine. They performed stress management activities, including deep breathing exercises and yoga. These practices helped them stay present, reduced anxiety, and enhanced their emotional connection.

Acknowledging that self-help had its limits, Mary and Jim decided to seek professional guidance. They connected with a therapist specializing in anxiety and stress management, a decision that transformed their approach to mental health. With the help of cognitive-behavioral therapy (CBT), they discovered effective techniques to cope with their anxiety. The combination of professional guidance, relaxation techniques, and the unconditional love of their pet empowered them to regain emotional balance and reduce their anxiety.

Key Lessons:

- **The Power of a Pet:** Mary and Jim found that bringing a dog into their lives provided comfort, companionship, and emotional support, helping them cope with anxiety and feel more grounded.

- **Relaxation Techniques Matter:** Practicing deep breathing and yoga helped Mary and Jim stay present, reduce stress, and strengthen their emotional connection.

- **Don't Hesitate to Seek Help:** When they realized self-help wasn't enough, Mary and Jim reached out to a therapist, gaining valuable tools and strategies to manage their anxiety more effectively.

Sleep Your Way to Better Sex

Quality sleep becomes even more important as you age, playing a key role in maintaining your overall health and sexual well-being. Lack of sleep can lead to lower energy, reduced libido, and even impact your mood. Here's why sleep is so essential for you:

- **Hormone Regulation:** Adequate sleep helps balance your hormones—testosterone and estrogen. Lack of sleep can cause imbalances, leading to reduced sexual desire and performance.

- **Physical Health:** Quality sleep is vital for physical health, lowering the risk of chronic conditions like diabetes, heart disease, and obesity. These health issues can negatively impact your sexual health and stamina.

- **Mental Health:** Sleep is vital for maintaining cognitive health by reducing stress, anxiety, and depression. Poor sleep can lead to a decline in mental well-being, which can affect your sexual desire and performance.

- **Energy Levels:** Ample sleep replenishes your energy levels. Enough rest can boost your energy and vitality, contributing to greater health and sexual satisfaction.

- **Cognitive Function:** Sleeping well improves mental functions like focus, memory, and mood. Better cognitive function can enhance communication and emotional intimacy with your partner, which are critical to a healthy sexual relationship.

- **Immune System Support:** Sufficient sleep strengthens your immune system, making you less likely to get sick. A robust immune system helps you stay healthy and enjoy an active sex life.

- **Circadian Rhythms:** Good sleep helps maintain regular circadian rhythms—essential for bodily functions. Disrupted sleep patterns can decrease libido and lead to sexual dysfunction.

Tips:

- **Prioritize Self-Care:** Engage in activities that bring you joy, whether it's a favorite hobby, spending time outdoors, or simply relaxing with a good book. Incorporating relaxation techniques like deep breathing or guided imagery can improve mood, reduce stress, and positively impact sexual health. Don't forget the importance of a good night's sleep—self-care isn't an indulgence. It's a crucial part of your overall wellness.

- **Seek Professional Support:** Stay connected with healthcare providers, therapists, or counselors who can help guide you through any physical or emotional challenges. Whether managing stress, addressing health concerns, or getting advice on sexual wellness, professional support can offer valuable tools and resources to keep you feeling your best.

CHAPTER 10

Bedroom Boosters

"Viagra is like Disneyland.
You wait an hour for a two-minute ride."
— Robin Williams, American Actor

Hormone Hang-Ups

Over time, your body experiences natural shifts in hormone levels. These essential hormones, pivotal in boosting energy, stabilizing mood, and supporting a healthy sex drive, gradually begin to decline. This can lead to noticeable effects on your health—physically, mentally, and sexually. You might experience lower libido, mood swings, changes in weight, or difficulty sleeping. Understanding how these hormonal shifts impact your overall well-being and sexual health is essential as you navigate aging. With the right knowledge and approach, you can take steps to maintain a healthy, active, and fulfilling life at every stage.

Fortunately, several treatment options are available to help manage the effects of hormonal changes. Hormone replacement therapy (HRT) is one option that can help balance declining levels of estrogen or testosterone, improving energy, mood, and sexual health. In addition to HRT, lifestyle changes like regular exercise, a balanced diet, and stress management can support your overall well-being. Natural supplements, certain medications, and alternative therapies such as acupuncture or herbal remedies can also be helpful.

Women and Menopause

Menopause marks an important phase in a woman's life, ending her reproductive years and bringing about a variety of physical and emotional changes. During this time, estrogen therapy (ET) and estrogen-progestogen therapy (EPT) play key roles in hormone replacement therapy (HRT). These treatments provide much-needed relief from common symptoms such as hot flashes and mood swings while also helping to prevent bone loss and reduce the risk of osteoporosis.

ET and EPT can ease the discomfort of menopause, making the transition smoother, by helping to restore hormonal balance. These therapies offer flexibility, allowing you to choose the best method for your health goals and lifestyle.

Men and Andropause

As men age, they will experience andropause, often called "low T," which presents its own set of challenges. Lower testosterone levels can lead to decreased sex drive, reduced muscle mass, and more frequent mood swings. Aging can sometimes require additional support, and this is where testosterone replacement therapy (TRT) comes into play.

TRT works by replenishing testosterone levels, helping to tackle issues like fatigue, low libido, erectile dysfunction (ED), depression, muscle loss, and even the risk of osteoporosis. It's a way to restore sexual vitality and energy. TRT offers several treatment options, allowing you to choose the method that fits your health needs.

Benefits of HRT

- **Relief from Symptoms:** Hormone replacement therapy (HRT) offers relief from the challenges that arise from hormonal changes. For women, it can ease common menopausal symptoms like hot flashes, night sweats, vaginal dryness, mood swings, and sleep disturbances. For men, HRT can help manage symptoms of andropause, including low testosterone, which can affect energy levels, mood, and sexual performance.

- **Bone Health:** Hormonal treatments can play a crucial role in preserving the strength of your bones as you age. In women, the natural drop in estrogen after menopause often leads to fragile bones and a higher risk of osteoporosis. For men, testosterone helps keep bones resilient and strong. Supporting your body's ability to maintain bone density can help prevent bone loss and reduce the likelihood of fracture.

- **Cardiovascular Health:** Hormonal balance also influences the heart and blood vessels. Restoring hormone levels can promote healthier cholesterol balances and potentially lower the risk of heart disease.

- **Mood and Cognitive Function:** Managing hormonal changes can improve mood, reduce anxiety and depression, and enhance mental clarity. Whether you're navigating menopause or andropause, these treatments help support emotional well-being and cognitive function.

- **Sexual Health:** Hormone therapy can address common sexual health concerns related to aging, such as low libido, sexual performance issues, and discomfort.

- **Quality of Life:** HRT can help smooth the transition through menopause or andropause, improving overall well-being and quality of life.

HRT – The Risks Revealed

- **Side Effects:** Some individuals may experience bloating, breast tenderness, headaches, or mood swings. These symptoms vary from person to person, and it's important to monitor how your body responds to treatment.

- **Cardiovascular Risks:** Hormonal therapies can increase the chance of developing blood clots, stroke, or heart disease, especially for individuals with pre-existing health conditions.

- **Gallbladder Disease:** Hormonal therapies, particularly estrogen-based treatments, have been associated with an increased risk of gallbladder disease. This is especially relevant for women undergoing estrogen therapy, as it may contribute to the formation of gallstones.

- **Liver Function:** Oral hormone treatments can impact liver function, particularly those containing estrogen. As the liver processes these hormones, it may experience added strain, affecting its ability to function optimally.

- **High Blood Pressure:** Hormonal treatments can elevate blood pressure, making regular monitoring essential during therapy.

- **Endometrial Cancer:** For women with a uterus, estrogen-only therapies can increase the risk of developing endometrial cancer. Adding progesterone lowers this risk, as progesterone helps balance the effects of estrogen on the uterine lining.

- **Other Cancers:** Prolonged use of hormone therapy, especially estrogen-progesterone combinations (EPT), may increase the risk of certain cancers, such as breast and ovarian cancer, for women. Men on long-term testosterone therapy should also be cautious, as there is a potential link to an increased risk of prostate cancer.

- **Mental Health Changes:** Hormonal treatments can influence mood and mental health. While some people experience improved emotional balance, others may notice increased anxiety, irritability, or depression.

Hormone therapy offers significant benefits and potential risks, making it important to tailor treatment to your unique needs. Personalizing HRT involves creating a treatment plan that fits your health history, age, and wellness goals. The aim is to enhance the positive effects, such as improved mood, bone health, and sexual well-being, while minimizing risks like cardiovascular issues or certain cancers. Open communication with your healthcare provider is crucial to ensure you make informed decisions and manage potential side effects. Ongoing research continues to refine our understanding and strategies for treating age-related hormone loss.

Case History: Frank and Sally's Rollercoaster

I crossed paths with Frank and Sally during my initial visit to The Villages. They were my temporary "neighbors" while I was there collecting data for my doctoral dissertation. From the moment we met, their genuine warmth and openness captivated me, and they eagerly shared their life experiences, making me feel right at home. As a college student, I certainly couldn't resist the bonus of delicious home-cooked meals, which deepened our connection.

Frank, a retired engineer in his early 60s, was grappling with the common signs of andropause—low energy, loss of muscle mass, and decreased libido. He also faced mood swings and persistent fatigue, which disrupted his daily routine and sense of well-being. After consulting with his doctor, Frank opted for TRT, choosing the injectable form as the most convenient option. Within a few months, the changes were striking. His energy surged, he regained muscle mass, and his libido returned. Emotionally, he felt more balanced, allowing him to fully re-engage with the activities he loved, including golf and volunteering.

Sally, a retired teacher in her late 50s, struggled with common menopause symptoms like hot flashes, night sweats, and a general decline in her sense of well-being. Despite these challenges, Sally was cautious about starting HRT due to concerns about the potential risks. Instead, she chose a more natural approach, focusing on a phytoestrogen-rich diet, regular exercise, and meditation. She took herbal supplements, such as black cohosh and red clover, known for their potential to alleviate menopausal discomfort. Sally also joined a support group for women experiencing menopause, where she gained valuable information and received emotional support.

Over time, Sally noticed that her symptoms became more manageable. Although the holistic approach didn't offer the rapid relief that some women find with HRT, she appreciated the steady, gradual improvements. This approach allowed her to feel more in control of her health, and her dedication to a healthier lifestyle left her feeling more energized and vibrant.

Key Lessons:

- **Personalize Health Treatments:** Frank and Sally's experiences show that health treatments should be customized to fit individual needs. Frank benefited from testosterone replacement therapy (TRT), while Sally thrived with a holistic approach. Their stories emphasize that no one-size-fits-all solution exists—explore different options and choose what works best for you.

- **Commit to Ongoing Monitoring:** Frank and Sally understood the value of regular health check-ins. Frank needed consistent follow-ups to keep his testosterone levels balanced, and Sally adjusted her holistic routine based on how her body responded. Continuous monitoring is essential for optimizing your health.

- **Build a Support System:** Frank found balance through TRT, golf, and volunteering, while Sally relied on her support network for emotional and practical help. Their experiences show the power of having a strong community, highlighting how essential support systems are when facing health challenges.

HRT Alternatives

It's important to understand your options when dealing with hormonal changes. While hormone replacement therapy (HRT) is a well-known choice, it's not your only option. Non-hormonal medications can address sexual dysfunction through different pathways, offering an effective alternative. If you're looking for a more permanent solution, surgical options can directly correct specific issues.

For those who prefer a natural approach, alternative therapies provide holistic methods to support and improve sexual health. These can include dietary supplements, acupuncture, herbal remedies, and lifestyle changes to help balance your body's natural systems. Explore what works best for you based on your preferences and needs.

Non-Hormonal Options

For women experiencing hypoactive sexual desire disorder (HSDD), which includes issues like low sexual desire, difficulty with arousal, problems with achieving orgasm, or pain during intercourse (dyspareunia)—there are effective non-hormonal treatment options available:

- **Flibanserin (Addyi):** This daily oral medication is designed to boost sexual desire by adjusting neurotransmitter levels in the brain. It's especially helpful for premenopausal women who have experienced low sexual desire that's led to emotional distress or relationship challenges. By rebalancing mood and desire-related chemicals, Flibanserin gradually improves sexual interest over time.

- **Bremelanotide (Vyleesi):** This is an on-demand treatment that's self-administered by injection about 45 minutes before anticipated sexual activity. It stimulates specific brain pathways related to sexual desire, providing a quick response. Unlike daily medications, Bremelanotide is ideal for those seeking flexibility, as it can be used only when needed.

For men experiencing erectile dysfunction (ED), which includes symptoms such as premature ejaculation, reduced sexual arousal, and low libido—there are several non-hormonal treatments to consider:

- **Oral Medications:** Oral medications are a common and effective treatment option for men with ED. Drugs such as Sildenafil (Viagra), Tadalafil (Cialis), Vardenafil (Levitra), and Avanafil (Stendra) help increase blood flow to the penis, making it easier to achieve and sustain an erection during sexual activity.

- **Alprostadil:** This medication offers a range of non-oral treatments for ED and can be administered in different forms based on personal preference and needs. Caverject is injected directly into the penis to enhance blood flow and achieve an erection. Muse is inserted into the urethra to improve circulation for improved erectile function. Vitaros is a topical cream applied directly to the penis, offering an easy-to-use alternative that helps boost blood flow and improve erections without the need for pills or injections. These options provide flexibility for men seeking non-oral treatment approaches for ED.

> *In The Villages, retirement is more than just golf and afternoon tea—it's a place where passion and friendly competition thrive!*
> *In fact, 34% of men use sexual performance-enhancing medications to keep the spark alive. And it's not just the men—19% of women also use similar aids, proving that passion has no expiration date.*
> *These retirees are redefining what it means to grow older, showing a bold commitment to staying vibrant and keeping the flames of passion burning!*

Surgical Breakthroughs

Surgical treatments for sexual dysfunction can be a transformative option, particularly when other medical or alternative therapies have not been effective. These procedures directly address the physical causes of sexual dysfunction, offering a long-term and often more reliable solution. Whether you're dealing with conditions like ED, Peyronie's disease, or HSDD—

surgical interventions have the potential to improve sexual function and well-being.

Surgical Options for Women

Women have access to a variety of surgical procedures specifically designed to address sexual dysfunction. These procedures can reduce discomfort, boost confidence in intimate relationships, and enhance overall sexual satisfaction. The following surgeries provide a pathway to improved sexual function, helping women experience a better quality of life.

Vaginoplasty

Vaginoplasty is a surgical procedure designed to tighten the vaginal canal, often performed after childbirth. During the surgery, excess vaginal lining is removed, and the surrounding tissues are tightened to restore tone and firmness. The benefits may include increased friction during intercourse, improved urinary control, and enhanced sexual satisfaction.

Labiaplasty

Labiaplasty reduces the size of the labia minora, the inner lips of the vulva. Women who experience discomfort or self-consciousness due to enlarged or asymmetrical labia often choose this procedure. Labiaplasty trims excess tissue and reshapes the labia minora, achieving a more symmetrical and aesthetically pleasing appearance. Besides cosmetic benefits, it can also reduce physical discomfort during activities like exercise or sexual intercourse, improving sexual confidence.

Clitoral Hood Reduction

Clitoral hood reduction is a surgical procedure that removes excess skin around the clitoris, which can reduce sensitivity. By uncovering more of the clitoris, this procedure can increase sexual sensation and make it easier to respond to stimulation. With less tissue blocking sensitivity, many women experience heightened sexual pleasure and greater overall satisfaction.

G-Shot

The G-shot, also known as G-spot amplification, is a cosmetic procedure where a dermal filler is injected into the front wall of the vagina near the G-spot. The goal is to enlarge and increase sensitivity in the area, potentially making it more responsive during sexual activity. Some women report enhanced sexual satisfaction and arousal after the procedure, though results vary from person to person.

Surgical Options for Men

Men have a variety of surgical treatments available to address sexual dysfunction, with each option designed to target specific underlying causes. The following surgical procedures provide options to help restore and improve sexual function to boost sexual health and satisfaction.

Inflatable Implants

Inflatable implants are a modern, effective solution for ED. The procedure involves placing fluid-filled cylinders inside the penis, which are connected to a small pump implanted in the scrotum. By activating the pump, the cylinders inflate, allowing the user to control both the timing and duration of the erection. When not in use, the cylinders can be deflated, maintaining the penis's natural look and feel. This option provides both spontaneity and discretion, offering a more natural and satisfying sexual experience.

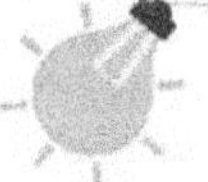

Malleable Implants

Malleable implants are a durable alternative to inflatable models, consisting of bendable rods that are surgically implanted into the erectile tissue of the penis. These rods can be manually positioned to achieve a firm state suitable for sexual intercourse. Malleable implants offer a simple and reliable solution for ED, particularly for individuals who have not found success with other treatments. They enable the maintenance of a firm erection when needed, significantly improving sexual function and boosting confidence.

Penile Vascular Reconstructive Surgery

Penile vascular reconstructive surgery is a specialized procedure designed to treat ED caused by blocked or damaged blood vessels in the penis. The surgery involves repairing existing blood vessels or bypassing them using grafts or implants to restore proper blood flow. This enhanced circulation improves erectile function, allowing for the achievement and maintenance of erections suitable for sexual activity, which can lead to improved sexual performance.

Varicocele Repair

Varicoceles are enlarged veins in the scrotum that can cause discomfort and negatively impact fertility by impairing sperm production. Varicocele repair is a surgical procedure that corrects this condition by tying off the swollen veins and redirecting blood flow through healthier vessels. This process helps reduce swelling and pain, improving sperm quality and fertility. Varicocele repair enhances comfort and supports reproductive health by relieving congestion in the scrotal veins.

Holistic Remedies

As you navigate the aging process, there are many natural alternatives to hormone replacement therapy (HRT), medications, or surgery. Holistic approaches offer effective ways to support sexual health and overall well-being. Techniques such as mindfulness, meditation, acupuncture, and the use of herbal supplements can make a noticeable difference. These methods work together to promote balance and vitality, enhancing sexual health while contributing to a greater quality of life. The following are some natural strategies for maintaining optimal health as you age.

Mindfulness and Meditation

Mindfulness and meditation are powerful techniques for improving sexual health. They help reduce stress and increase awareness of your body and mind. This allows you to connect more deeply with your physical sensations and emotional states. Techniques like deep breathing, progressive muscle relaxation, and guided imagery are particularly effective for promoting relaxation and presence.

Benefits of Mindfulness and Meditation

- **Reduced Stress and Anxiety:** Mindfulness and meditation can alleviate performance anxiety and boost sexual desire by calming your mind and lowering physiological stress responses.

- **Improved Mental Clarity:** These practices help clear mental clutter, allowing you to focus more fully on your partner and the sexual experience, enhancing intimacy and connection.

- **Stronger Mind-Body Connection:** Heightened awareness of bodily sensations and emotional states can lead to more satisfying sexual encounters and increased arousal.

- **Enhanced Sexual Experiences:** Mindfulness encourages you to tune into your sexual desires and responses, resulting in a more fulfilling and satisfying sexual life.

Acupuncture

Acupuncture is an ancient Chinese practice that involves inserting thin needles into specific points on your body to balance your energy flow. It can enhance sexual function by addressing issues like hormonal imbalances, stress, and poor circulation.

Benefits of Acupuncture

- **Improved Blood Flow:** Acupuncture can enhance blood circulation, which is crucial for sexual arousal and performance.

- **Hormonal Balance:** This practice can help regulate hormones, potentially improving libido and sexual function.

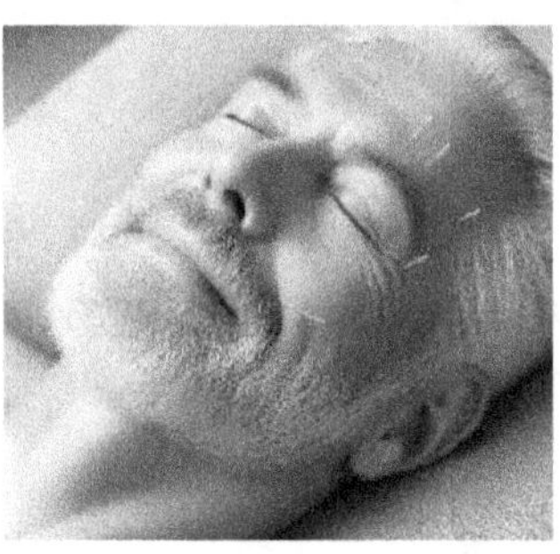

- **Stress Reduction:** Acupuncture is known for its ability to reduce stress and promote relaxation, contributing to a better overall sexual experience.

Herbal Supplements

Herbal supplements can provide a natural way to support sexual health and well-being, especially among older adults. Beyond the popular options of maca root and ginseng covered in Chapter 7, other herbal supplements include Tribulus terrestris, horny goat weed, ginkgo biloba, ashwagandha, fenugreek, and damiana.

Benefits of Herbal Supplements

- **Increased Libido:** Certain herbs are known to naturally enhance sexual desire and boost energy levels, helping to reignite passion and intimacy.

- **Enhanced Stamina:** Many herbal supplements can improve endurance, allowing for greater stamina—contributing to a more satisfying sexual life.

- **Overall Wellness Boost:** Herbal remedies often help elevate mood, reduce stress, and increase vitality, promoting a healthier, more balanced lifestyle.

Tips:

- **Consider Hormone Replacement Therapy:** HRT can improve your sexual health by alleviating troublesome symptoms. Weigh the pros and cons carefully and discuss whether HRT aligns with your needs and lifestyle.

- **Explore Holistic Alternatives:** If HRT isn't right for you, there are other options to support your sexual health and vitality. Consider holistic methods like mindfulness and meditation, acupuncture, and herbal supplements.

CHAPTER 11

Talk It Out and Love It Up

"Sex is not just about pleasure; it's about communication,
intimacy, and connection."

— Shirley MacLaine, American Actress

Breaking the Silence

Communication is key to building and maintaining strong relationships, helping you share your thoughts, feelings, and needs with others. As you age, you may face new challenges that make communication harder, such as hearing loss, memory changes, or a natural decline in speech. Medications and health issues can also affect how clearly you think and express yourself. These difficulties can have a big impact on your sexual health and intimacy since open and honest communication is crucial for sharing desires and staying emotionally connected. Understanding how communication changes as you age can help you maintain satisfying relationships. Here are some simple strategies to overcome communication challenges and deepen your connection with your partner.

Address Hearing Loss

- **Use Hearing Aids:** If you experience hearing loss, using hearing aids can greatly improve your ability to stay engaged in conversations, including intimate discussions with your partner. This helps you remain connected and involved.

- **Encourage Clear Communication:** Ask your partner to speak clearly and at a steady pace, making it easier for you to follow conversations. Patience and thoughtful communication improve understanding and strengthen your emotional connection, making both of you feel more valued.

Enhance Cognitive Function

- **Keep Your Mind Active:** Engage in activities that challenge your brain, such as puzzles, reading, or learning new skills. Staying mentally sharp helps you think clearly and communicate more effectively.

- **Eat a Brain-Healthy Diet:** A balanced diet rich in nutrients supports your brain health and keeps your mind sharp, making it easier to have meaningful conversations and stay mentally alert.

Overcome Physical Barriers

- **Manage Your Medications:** If certain medications affect your focus or mental clarity, talk to your doctor. Adjusting or finding alternatives can improve how well you think and communicate.

- **Stay Physically Active:** Regular exercise benefits both your body and mind. It boosts your overall health and energy, helping you communicate more easily and clearly.

Combat Social Isolation

- **Stay Connected with Others:** Make an effort to keep in touch with friends, family, and your community. Participating in social activities can enrich your life and improve your communication skills.

- **Find Support:** Joining support groups can provide companionship and shared experiences. Feeling connected to others enhances emotional well-being and helps you stay engaged in conversations.

Address Emotional Barriers

- **Seek Professional Support:** If you're dealing with anxiety, depression, or low self-esteem, it can impact your ability to communicate openly. Reaching out to a therapist or counselor can help you work through these challenges, improving both your emotional and sexual health.

- **Practice Opening Up:** Regularly sharing your thoughts and feelings with trusted friends or family helps you become more comfortable expressing yourself. Honest, open communication is the foundation of stronger, more fulfilling relationships.

Embrace Technology

- **Learn New Tech Skills:** Attend workshops in The Villages to learn how to use social media, messaging apps, or video calls. Being tech-savvy can help you stay connected with loved ones, boost emotional intimacy, and keep communication flowing.

- **Stay Informed:** Keep up with the latest communication tools to enhance your connections. Using technology to stay close to friends and family improves your overall well-being and supports a healthy and satisfying intimate life.

Intimacy Unplugged

Intimacy is the foundation of deep, meaningful relationships, blending emotional closeness, physical affection, and shared moments. It's vital for creating a fulfilling partnership and maintaining a healthy, satisfying connection. Intimacy takes many forms—emotional, physical, social, intellectual, and spiritual. Each type adds its own unique layer of depth, helping you and your partner grow closer and more connected over time. By nurturing these different

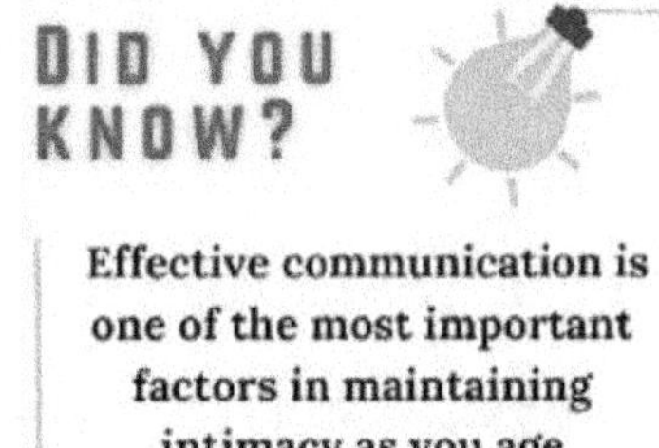

forms of intimacy, you build a stronger, more resilient relationship that thrives on trust, understanding, and shared experiences.

Emotional Intimacy

- **Share Openly:** Express your thoughts, feelings, and vulnerabilities with your partner. Being open creates trust and creates a safe space for emotional closeness and deeper connection.

- **Listen Actively:** When your partner is speaking, give them your full attention. Show empathy, avoid interruptions, and make them feel truly heard and valued. This helps strengthen your emotional bond.

Physical Intimacy

- **Show Affection:** Simple gestures like holding hands, hugging, or sharing a kiss can go a long way in maintaining physical closeness and affection throughout the day. These small acts reinforce your connection.

- **Build Trust:** Trust is the foundation of physical intimacy. Make sure both you and your partner feel safe, comfortable, and respected in each other's presence, allowing intimacy to grow naturally.

Social Intimacy

- **Explore New Experiences:** Try new things together, like picking up a new hobby or introducing fresh ideas into your relationship. This adds excitement and strengthens your connection.

- **Create Rituals:** Establish regular routines, like sharing a morning coffee, taking evening walks, or setting aside time for weekly date nights. These simple, consistent practices help you build emotional closeness.

Intellectual Intimacy

- **Engage in Stimulating Conversations:** Have meaningful discussions on topics that interest both of you. Sharing your thoughts, exchanging ideas, and learning creates a deeper intellectual connection.

- **Collaborate on Problem-Solving:** Tackle challenges or make decisions as a team. Whether solving puzzles, planning for the future, or working through tasks, this collaborative effort strengthens your intellectual bond.

Spiritual Intimacy

- **Share Your Values and Beliefs:** Open up about your personal values, beliefs, and life goals. Whether these are related to faith or general principles, aligning on them can deepen your spiritual connection and bring you closer.

- **Practice Mindfulness:** Engage in mindfulness or meditation practices as a couple. These activities encourage peace, reflection, and unity, helping you connect on a more profound spiritual level.

Building Stronger Bonds

Maintaining a solid connection with your partner is crucial for a healthy and fulfilling relationship, especially as you transition into retirement. After years of focusing on work, raising children, and managing the daily hustle, retirement offers the gift of time—time to truly enjoy each other's company, reconnect, and rediscover intimacy. This phase of life can deepen emotional closeness, as you're no longer juggling competing priorities. Instead, you have the opportunity to focus on nurturing your relationship.

Having more time together allows for shared activities and meaningful conversations, which can help rekindle feelings of love and closeness. Whether taking long walks, cooking meals, traveling, engaging in hobbies, or simply having quiet moments together, these shared experiences can strengthen your bond. The reduced stress that comes with retirement can also lead to improved physical health, allowing for more energy and vitality in your relationship. These benefits extend to your sexual life, where open communication, relaxation, and a stronger emotional connection can lead to more fulfilling intimate experiences.

Be Supportive

Being a supportive partner is essential in fostering a deep, lasting connection, especially during life's highs and lows. Your encouragement and understanding provide a foundation of emotional security that can positively impact your partner's well-being. During challenging times, whether they're facing health issues, emotional stress, or personal setbacks, your presence and compassion can help them feel valued and understood. This emotional support strengthens your bond, creating a safe space for vulnerability and openness.

Support doesn't just come in times of struggle; it's also about celebrating your partner's achievements, joys, and growth. Being present, actively listening, and showing genuine interest in their experiences establishes a sense of mutual respect and appreciation that enhances emotional closeness. This emotional intimacy naturally carries over into your physical relationship, as feeling emotionally secure and supported can deepen trust and allow for a more fulfilling and connected intimate life. Here are some ways to offer your partner support:

- **Listen Without Judgement:** Sometimes, simply listening to your partner's concerns or frustrations without offering immediate solutions can provide the understanding they need.

- **Show Empathy:** Acknowledge their feelings and experiences, even if you may not fully understand them. This empathy enables a sense of closeness and validation.

- **Offer Reassurance:** During difficult times, remind your partner that you're a team and that you're in this together. Knowing they have someone to lean on can relieve stress and create a stronger connection.

- **Celebrate Their Wins:** Don't overlook the importance of celebrating the good times. Being supportive means recognizing your partner's successes and sharing their happiness, reinforcing positivity in your relationship.

- **Be Patient:** Patience during tough moments is key. Whether recovering from a health issue or navigating emotional challenges, offering steady, calm support helps create a nurturing environment where intimacy can thrive.

- **Keep the Romance Alive:** Surprise your partner with small gestures of love, such as date nights, thoughtful gifts, or heartfelt notes. Keeping the romance alive adds excitement and joy to your relationship, enhancing intimacy and overall satisfaction.

> *Insights from The Villages' residents show that 93% believe that flirtation and playful teasing add extra excitement to their intimate lives. These small acts of romance help keep relationships fresh and fun! Many couples maintain closeness through physical touch, with 61% of men and 53% of women enjoying things like foot rubs and back massages more than once a week. However, not everyone engages as often—20% of men and 15% of women say they experience this kind of mutual caressing just 1-3 times a year, and for 18% of women and 8% of men, it's even rarer. Here's to more back rubs and foot massages to keep the romance alive and thriving!*

Tips:

- **Communicate Openly with Your Partner:** Good communication is essential for a satisfying, intimate life. Talk openly with your partner about your needs, desires, and concerns. Honest conversations help you both feel more connected and make your sexual experiences more enjoyable and fulfilling.

- **Keep Intimacy Alive in Simple Ways:** Intimacy goes beyond physical pleasure—it's about deep connection and emotional closeness. Strengthen your bond by spending quality time together in small, meaningful ways. Hold hands while walking, enjoy long hugs, or cuddle on the couch while watching a movie. Even quiet moments shared in comfortable silence can create a sense of togetherness.

CHAPTER 12

Silver Screen Romance

---

*"You're never too old to set another goal or to dream a new dream—
even if that dream is love."*

— C.S. Lewis, British Author

Relationships in Retirement

One of the great advantages of dating in retirement is the freedom to explore new relationships without the constraints of career obligations or family duties. With this stage of life comes the luxury of time—time to indulge in romantic getaways, discover new hobbies, and truly enjoy each other's company. It's a unique chapter where personal happiness and deep emotional connections take center stage, paving the way for more meaningful and fulfilling relationships. Embrace this newfound freedom and the exciting possibilities that come with it!

Dating and romance in The Villages can be just as exhilarating and fulfilling as they were in your younger years. Whether looking for new companionship or aiming to keep the spark alive, this vibrant retirement community offers plenty of opportunities for love and connection. Community activities, clubs, and social events create perfect settings for meaningful relationships. There are numerous ways to meet like-minded individuals who share your interests and zest for life, from salsa dance classes and wine-tasting events to community theatre productions.

Whether single, divorced, or widowed, The Villages offers a dynamic dating scene where companionship and romance are always within reach. The community's lively atmosphere makes it easy to meet new people and form connections that can enhance your overall happiness.

Swipe Right Like a Pro

In The Villages, where social activities are abundant, residents seek more than just casual friendships—they seek profound, personal connections. While traditional pastimes like clubs, dances, and community events continue attracting residents, many older adults are turning to online dating to find companionship and romance. Combating loneliness and establishing meaningful connections are top priorities, and online dating has transformed how people seek and build romantic relationships.

Studies show that older adults are becoming more comfortable using the internet and mobile apps for dating and meeting new people. According to the Pew Research Center, over 20% of adults aged 55–64 have tried dating apps, as did 13% of adults aged 64 and older. Other research identified an overall trend of gender differences in online dating among adults aged 60 and older. Men were significantly more likely to participate in online dating compared to women. Women sought an honest partner who would participate in leisure activities with them. In contrast, men sought physically attractive women who would provide emotional support.

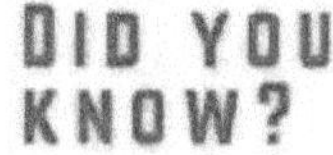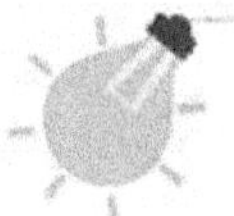

Many older adults report successful relationships formed through online dating

Online dating sites are designed to be simple and easy to use, especially for those who may find traditional dating methods challenging. If you're ready to step into a new way of meeting people, here are some reasons why online dating could be for you:

- **Expand Your Horizons:** Online dating lets you connect with potential partners beyond your immediate community. This broader reach increases your chances of finding someone who matches your interests and values.

- **Embrace Flexibility and Convenience:** You can explore profiles and engage in conversations at your own pace from the comfort of your computer. This flexibility makes it easier to fit dating into your daily routine.

- **Meet Like-Minded Individuals:** Online dating platforms often use algorithms to match you with individuals who share similar interests and goals. This increases the likelihood of forming meaningful connections that lead to long-term, fulfilling relationships.

- **Overcome Physical Barriers:** If mobility is an issue, online dating eliminates the need for extensive travel. You can meet new people and build relationships without leaving your home, making connecting with others and maintaining an active romantic life easier.

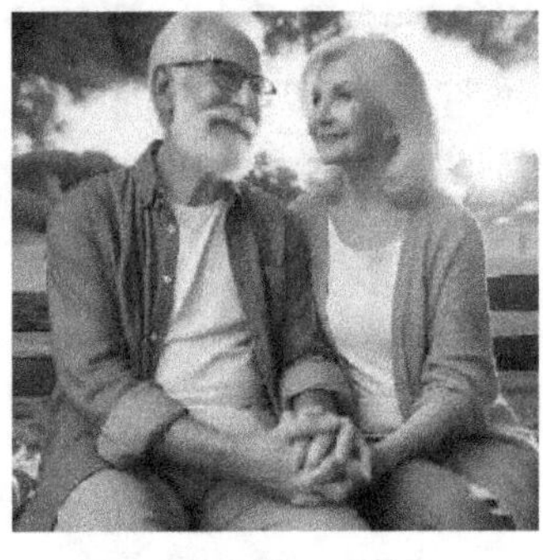

Steps for Digital Dating

In The Villages, many residents embrace the digital age by using dating apps and online platforms tailored to the 50+ community. These tools offer an exciting way to meet new people, explore potential relationships, and enhance your social life. If you're considering dating online, here are some practical steps to ensure your experience is successful and enjoyable.

1. Choose the Right Platform

Select a dating site or app that caters specifically to older adults. Platforms like OurTime, SilverSingles, and SeniorMatch are designed for the 50+ community and offer features that meet your unique needs and preferences. These platforms provide a comfortable and tailored experience, making it easier to find meaningful connections with like-minded individuals.

2. Create an Authentic Profile

Your dating profile serves as your first impression, making it essential to present yourself in a genuine and appealing way. To attract meaningful connections, focus on creating a profile showcasing who you truly are and what you seek in a partner.

- **Use Recent Photos:** Posting clear, recent photos is crucial. Choose images that reflect your true appearance and lifestyle, highlighting moments that reveal your personality. Whether it's a photo of you enjoying a hobby, spending time outdoors, or at a social event, authentic images offer a glimpse into your life and help potential matches get a sense of who you are. Avoid heavily edited or outdated photos, which can create a misleading first impression.

- **Write a Compelling Bio:** Your bio is your chance to tell your story. Focus on sharing your values, interests, and what you want in a partner. Mentioning your hobbies and passions makes you more relatable while highlighting unique aspects of your personality can set you apart. A well-crafted bio offers potential matches insight into what drives you and what you value most in life. Be specific about the qualities you seek in a relationship, but also leave room for curiosity and discovery.

- **Be Honest:** Honesty is the foundation of any successful relationship, so being truthful about your age, interests, and intentions is essential. Authenticity helps build trust, which in turn attracts connections that align with your goals. Whether you're seeking friendship, companionship, or something long-term—clarity about your desires allows others to engage with you in a genuine way.

3. Prioritize Safety

While online dating provides a convenient way to meet new people, safeguarding your personal safety should always be a top priority. By taking thoughtful precautions, you can enjoy your dating experience with peace of mind.

- **Use Reputable Sites:** Stick to established, well-reviewed dating platforms prioritizing user security. These sites often have advanced privacy settings and verification processes that help protect users from scams or inappropriate behavior. Reading reviews or doing some research before signing up can help ensure you're joining a site with a solid reputation for safety.

- **Protect Personal Information:** Keeping personal information private when interacting with someone new is essential. Avoid sharing details such as your home address, financial information, or other identifying information that could compromise your privacy or safety. Early conversations should remain focused on getting to know each other without delving into private matters.

- **Meet in Public Places:** When transitioning from online interactions to in-person meetings, always choose a public location for the first few dates. This provides a neutral, safer space where you can feel comfortable and secure. Public places such as cafes, parks, or restaurants ensure a safer environment and allow you both to focus on enjoying each other's company without any pressure.

4. Engage Thoughtfully

When communicating with potential matches, keep these tips in mind:

- **Be Respectful:** Treat others with kindness and respect. Good manners go a long way in building a positive connection.

- **Take Your Time:** Don't rush into anything. Take the time to gradually get to know the person and let the relationship develop naturally.

- **Be Open:** Keep an open mind and be willing to explore different types of connections. You might be surprised by who you connect with and how relationships can evolve.

5. Enjoy The Process

- **Have Fun:** Approach dating with a positive attitude. Enjoy the process of meeting new people and discovering different personalities.

- **Stay Active:** Regularly check your messages and engage with those who reach out. Consistent activity increases your chances of finding meaningful connections.

- **Learn and Grow:** Each interaction is an opportunity to learn more about yourself and what you want in a relationship. Embrace the journey of self-discovery and personal growth.

6. Seek Support and Advice

Don't hesitate to seek support from friends or family who may have experience with online dating. Their insights can be invaluable:

- **Join a Group:** Consider joining a local or online group specifically for older adults exploring online dating. These communities provide valuable support, practical advice, and a sense of connection, helping you navigate the dating landscape with confidence.

- **Share Experiences:** Talk about your experiences and listen to others. Sharing stories and advice can provide encouragement and helpful tips, making your dating journey more enjoyable and less daunting.

Online dating offers a fantastic opportunity to enhance your social life and find meaningful connections. By choosing the right platform, creating an authentic profile, prioritizing safety, and engaging thoughtfully—you can make the most of your online dating experience. Remember, dating should be fun and fulfilling. Approach it with an open heart and a positive mindset, and you'll discover new opportunities for companionship and romance. Here are some handy "dos and don'ts" to steer you through your digital dating journey:

The Do's and Don'ts of Online Dating

1. **Do know what you're fishing for!** Grab a pen and write down your must-haves—honesty, emotional availability, respect, good communication, and mutual attraction. Then, make a list of your nice-to-haves—someone who can whip up a good meal, enjoys the same activities, loves to travel, or is handy around the house. Think of it like grocery shopping, but this time, you're shopping for love!

2. **Don't sink your ship!** Keep some mystery alive—there's no need to reveal all your secrets right away. Guard your privacy like it's the secret recipe for Coca-Cola!

3. **Do request a mugshot!** If their profile is missing a photo, don't be shy—ask for one. Stick to people with at least two or three recent snapshots. And while you're at it, upload at least two or three current pictures of yourself. Show off what you love—dining out, playing pickleball, painting, or boating. Just avoid anything too personal, like standing in front of your house. Keep it fun, not too revealing!

4. **Don't dive in headfirst!** Take your time and only meet when you're ready. If something seems too good to be true, it probably is. A healthy dose of caution and common sense will be your best allies here.

5. **Do chat on the phone!** Even better, try FaceTime for a little sneak preview. A simple phone call can speak volumes about someone—especially how well they communicate. If it's a flop, no worries! Swipe on to the next adventure.

6. **Don't ignore the red flags!** If they're avoiding a phone conversation before meeting, take that as a sign. Be cautious of anger or if they're pushing you into anything. And remember, consistency is key—if their story doesn't quite add up, it's best to move on.

7. **Do practice safety!** Always meet in a public place for your first date and be sure to inform a friend or family member about your plans. Avoid home pick-ups—keep things simple and secure. And dress well—first impressions matter, no matter what age we are.

8. **Don't get stranded!** Your safety is the top priority on a first date. Carry a fully charged phone, and if something doesn't feel right, trust your instincts and politely leave. No matter how charming your date is, avoid going to their place afterward—stay in control of your surroundings.

9. **Do cast your net wide!** If your date didn't spark a connection, don't worry! There are plenty of potential matches out there, whether locally or beyond. Keep looking, and don't settle for less than you deserve.

10. **Don't forget—you deserve a catch that makes you happy!** Take your time and find someone who truly brings joy and positivity into your life. You deserve a relationship that makes you happy, so be patient and enjoy the journey. Happy fishing!

Case History: George and Linda's Romance

Life in The Villages is always filled with delightful surprises and chance encounters. One memorable evening, I crossed paths with George and Linda during a leisurely stroll.

George, a charismatic salesman with a mischievous grin, welcomed me with a playful, "Third time's the charm, right?" referring to his two previous marriages and the joy of raising three wonderful children. Linda, on the other hand, was newly retired and navigating her independence after losing her husband. Eager to explore the dating world, she met George through an online dating site.

Their first meeting was a perfect reflection of their personalities. "When I saw her profile, I thought, 'She's way out of my league,'" George confessed with a grin. Linda, however, was instantly charmed by his candid, self-deprecating humor. "He's got that whole bad dad joke thing going on," she laughed, "but it's oddly endearing."

Their first date was filled with both nervous energy and genuine excitement. George captivated Linda with lighthearted stories from his life as a father. "I once fixed a Barbie dream house with nothing but duct tape and a prayer," he quipped proudly, to which Linda responded with warm laughter—they quickly found themselves bantering like old friends.

As their relationship deepened, so did their openness about more serious topics like sexual health. George, having faced life's ups and downs, spoke candidly about the physical and emotional challenges he has encountered. "It's not just about being physically ready," he remarked with a mix of humor and sincerity, "it's about being physically prepared."

George approached the topic of sexual performance with his trademark humor. "Well, this isn't my first challenge, but it's definitely my first time dealing with ED," he quipped, lightening the mood as he sought medical advice. Linda, still adjusting to the complexities of a new relationship after being recently widowed, faced her own uncertainties but remained a source of unwavering support. "We're in this together," she reassured him with a smile.

For Linda, rediscovering intimacy after her loss was both thrilling and a bit daunting. "I'm not as young as I used to be," she laughed, as they found themselves exploring new ways to connect. "Who would've thought we'd be feeling like teenagers again?" Their shared openness and humor made navigating this new chapter not just possible, but deeply meaningful.

Key Lessons:

- **Have the Courage to Start Again:** George and Linda's story shows that it's never too late to begin anew. Despite George's past marriages and Linda's journey through grief after losing her husband, they both found the strength to open their hearts again, demonstrating resilience and optimism.

- **Embrace Honesty and Vulnerability:** Open communication was key to their relationship, especially when discussing sensitive topics like sexual health and emotional readiness. Their willingness to be honest and vulnerable built a foundation of trust and strengthened their bond.

- **Offer Support and Mutual Respect:** George and Linda's relationship thrived because they supported each other's concerns with empathy and respect. By approaching challenges with care and understanding, they created a loving partnership that prioritized mutual growth and connection.

Single and Ready to Mingle?

You're in the right place! The Villages has an abundance of resources created just for its single residents, making it easy and fun to meet new people and maybe even find that special someone.

The Villages Singles Club and Straight Singles Club

If you're looking for social activities and opportunities to connect, these clubs have you covered. They organize regular events like singles' dance nights, mixers, and group dining—ideal for meeting new people in a relaxed, enjoyable setting. Whether you're dancing the night away or sharing stories over a delicious meal, you'll find yourself in the company of others who are just as excited to make new connections as you are! These events create a fun, low-pressure environment where friendships can blossom and, who knows, maybe even something more.

Speed Dating

If you like things a little more fast-paced, speed dating might be right up your alley! These events are popular among residents who want to meet a variety of people in a fun, structured setting. Keep an eye on community boards and club newsletters for upcoming dates— it's a great way to meet people who are also excited to find companionship, and you might be surprised at the sparks that fly!

Online Dating Workshops

The Villages offers valuable workshops designed for those ready to explore the world of online companionship or romance. These sessions provide expert advice on everything from navigating online dating platforms to crafting a profile that stands out. You'll also learn essential tips for safely meeting new people in the digital age—all without leaving the comfort of your community.

As online dating becomes more integrated into The Villages' social fabric, it offers endless possibilities for connection and companionship. The community's dynamic blend of traditional social activities and modern technology creates a supportive and exciting environment for finding love and friendship.

Participating in singles clubs, speed dating events, and online dating workshops can expand your social circle, opening the door to meaningful relationships. The Villages is committed to offering you the resources and opportunities needed to foster those connections, ensuring that your later years are filled with joy, companionship, and the possibility of love.

Tips:

- **Embrace Dating in Later Life:** It's never too late to dive back into the dating scene! Enjoy the process of meeting new people, forming connections, and letting relationships evolve naturally. Dating in your later years can be one of the most exciting and rewarding chapters of your life.

CHAPTER 13

Fantasies and Desires

"In a great romance, each person plays a part the other really likes."
— Elizabeth Ashley, American Actress

Sexual Fantasies and Desires

Your sexual fantasies—those private, unspoken daydreams—are a window into your deepest desires and can play a vital role in your well-being. As you grow older, your relationship with intimacy naturally evolves, much like other aspects of life. While some may believe that sexual desires fade with age, they often transform instead of disappearing. In fact, this stage of life can bring a greater awareness of your personal needs, a deeper sense of emotional intimacy, and a newfound appreciation for physical and emotional closeness.

Your fantasies might shift, becoming more emotionally driven, reflecting the wisdom and life experience you've gained. You may find yourself drawn to fantasies centered on connection, trust, and shared experiences rather than the thrill of novelty. Or, this could be a time when your curiosity encourages you to explore new fantasies, perhaps experimenting with sex toys or trying different sexual positions that bring fresh sensations and a renewed sense of excitement.

Embracing your desires can lead to deeper intimacy and a more fulfilling relationship with yourself and your partner. This chapter will help you understand the importance of these fantasies in your sexual health journey. Let's take a closer look at how fantasies and desires can enhance your overall well-being.

Role-Playing

Role-playing can be a fun and interactive way to explore new dynamics and deepen your connection with your partner. It involves taking on and acting out different roles or scenarios, which can add variety and excitement to your relationship. Here's how to get started:

- **Communicate Openly:** Talk with your partner about role-playing. Clear communication is critical to setting boundaries and understanding each other's preferences.

- **Choose a Scenario:** Pick a role-playing scenario that interests both of you. It could be something simple, like a romantic dinner date with a twist, or more adventurous, like exploring a fantasy world. Popular themes include historical eras, favorite movie characters, or everyday roles like a chef and a customer.

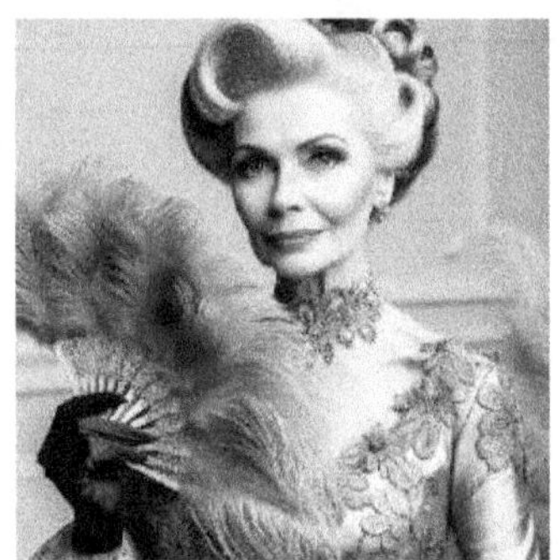

- **Set the Scene:** Create an environment that enhances the role-playing experience. Use props, costumes, or decorations to transform your space. For example, use beach towels, sunglasses, and a fruity drink if you're role-playing a beach scene.

- **Define Your Characters:** Give your characters names, backgrounds, and personalities. This adds depth and makes the role-playing more immersive. Have fun with it, and don't worry about being perfect.

- **Be Playful and Flexible:** Approach role-playing with a playful attitude. Things might not go exactly as planned, and that's okay. The goal is to enjoy each other's company and have fun exploring new dynamics.

- **Respect Boundaries:** Always respect each other's boundaries and comfort levels. If something feels uncomfortable, communicate openly and adjust as needed to ensure a safe and enjoyable experience.

- **Reflect and Share:** After the role-playing session, discuss what you enjoyed and might want to try next. Sharing your experiences helps improve future role-playing sessions and keeps the experience enjoyable.

Example Scenario

I. Scenario:

You and your partner pretend to meet at a restaurant as strangers. Choose a venue where you won't run into familiar faces. This playful scenario can set the stage for a romantic and memorable evening at home.

II. Setting:

Pick a lively restaurant that invites conversation. Dress elegantly to set the mood for an unforgettable night.

III. Roles:

- **Steven** is a charming and witty travel writer visiting the town, always equipped with captivating stories from distant lands.

- **Donna** is a retired art teacher with a deep passion for storytelling, eager to share tales of artistic adventures and creative journeys.

IV. Activities:

1. **The Encounter:**

   - **Steven** arrives first, sitting at the bar and reading the menu.

   - **Donna** enters shortly after, looking for a table, but heads toward the bar. With a flirtatious grin, Donna approaches Steven and asks, "Is this seat taken, or is it reserved for someone special?"

2. **The Introduction:**

   - **Steven** (extending a hand): "I'm Steven, a travel writer passing through. And you?"

   - **Donna** (shaking his hand): "Donna, a retired art teacher seeking new stories. Nice to meet you, Steven."

3. **The Banter:**

   o **Steven:** "So, Donna, what brings an art aficionado to this corner of the world?"

   o **Donna:** "Chasing inspiration and a bit of adventure. And you, Steven, find any good stories lately?"

   o **Steven:** "A few, but tonight's encounter might be the most interesting yet."

4. **The Flirtation:**

   o **Donna:** "Do you always charm strangers with tales of your travels?"

   o **Steven:** "Only the intriguing ones. And you, do you always captivate writers with your art?"

   o **Donna** (smirking): "Only the ones worth captivating."

5. **The Dinner:**

   o **Bartender:** "Are you ready to order?"

   o **Steven:** "I'll have the seafood special. How about you, Donna?"

   o **Donna:** "The pasta sounds perfect. Any wine recommendations?"

   o **Steven:** "A glass of the house red for both of us. It pairs well with good conversation."

6. **The Tease:**

   o **Donna:** "Maybe you can tell me more about that exotic beach in Bali after dinner."

   o **Steven:** "And perhaps you can show me some of your favorite art pieces back at your place."

7. **Exchange "Contact Info":**

    o   **Steven:** "This was fun, Donna. How about giving me your number so we can continue this sometime?"

    o   **Donna:** "Only if you promise more stories and maybe a visit to your favorite beach."

8. **Goodbye with a Hint:**

    o   **Donna:** "Tonight has been delightful, Steven. How about we take this conversation to my place? I have some art that might inspire your next story."

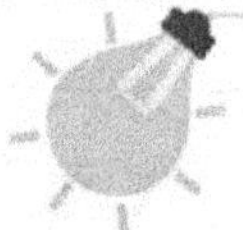

Role-playing allows older adults to explore new fantasies and desires, enhancing sexual satisfaction

    o   **Steven:** "Lead the way, Donna. I would love to see your art."

This playful scenario adds a spark of fun to your evening, setting the stage for a romantic and intimate night. The chemistry and banter between you and your partner will create a captivating vibe, catching the attention of those around you—even the bartender!

Solo Adventures in Self-Love

No partner? No problem! Let's explore a topic that often raises eyebrows—masturbation!

Masturbation isn't just a guilty pleasure—it's a healthy way to address your sexual needs. Research shows that solo sexual activities are essential for sexual satisfaction. It's about more than just physical pleasure; it's also about staying connected to your body and desires.

In The Villages, men and women show distinct differences when it comes to self-pleasure habits. For women, 63% reported not engaging in self-pleasure at all. Meanwhile, 12% indulged once a year, 18%

did so monthly, and only 7% enjoyed it weekly. Men, on the other hand, were more active in this area. While 41% abstained, 25% treated themselves once a year, 24% made it a monthly habit, and 10% engaged weekly.

This data sheds light on an often-private aspect of sexual health, revealing that men tend to practice self-pleasure more regularly than women. It provides a rare glimpse into how intimate habits continue to vary, even in later stages of life.

When physical intimacy isn't always possible, solo activities can be an important way to maintain a satisfying sex life. Masturbation offers several benefits that can enhance your physical and emotional wellness. Some of the key benefits include:

Health Benefits: Masturbation can help reduce stress, improve sleep, and boost mood. It's a natural way to maintain mental and physical well-being.

Self-Discovery: Exploring your body helps you understand what pleases you, making it easier to communicate your needs to a partner.

Independence: Solo activities allow you to fulfill your sexual needs without depending on someone, giving you a sense of autonomy and control.

Privacy: Engaging in solo sexual activities provides a private and intimate way to explore your desires without any pressure or judgment.

Enhanced Intimacy: Understanding your body can strengthen intimacy with a partner, as you can share what you've learned about your likes and dislikes.

Sexual Satisfaction: Solo play provides an outlet for sexual expression and satisfaction, especially for those who may not have a partner.

Tips:

- **Discover Your Fantasies Together**: Opening up about your sexual fantasies can bring a new level of excitement and intimacy to your relationship, helping you connect on a deeper level.

- **Introduce Role-Playing for Variety**: Role-playing can breathe fresh life into your intimate moments. Stepping into different roles allows you and your partner to explore new dynamics and enjoy the playful side of your relationship.

CHAPTER 14

Bedroom Toys

"Sex is something we can all learn from. A vibrator is something we can all learn with."

— Cynthia Heimel, American Author

Dare to Experiment

You may have heard about sex toys but never considered them for yourself. Perhaps the idea feels a bit unfamiliar, or maybe you're curious about how they work and what they could offer. Many older adults are discovering that sex toys can be a fun, safe way to enhance solo and partnered intimacy.

As we age, our sexual needs and preferences can shift. What brought you pleasure in your younger years may not have the same impact now. That's where sex toys can make a difference. They offer a way to reconnect with your body, enhance pleasure, and make intimacy more enjoyable—especially if you're experiencing changes like reduced sensitivity or a lower libido.

In this chapter, we'll explore the variety of sex toys available, how to choose one that suits your comfort level, and ways to use them that feel right for you. Whether you're looking to add excitement to your sex life or simply try something new, this guide will help you navigate your options with confidence.

Pleasure Parties

You might be surprised to learn that sex toy parties—or "pleasure parties" as they're often called—are becoming increasingly popular, especially among older adults looking to explore new ways to enhance their intimate lives. These gatherings offer a comfortable, social setting to learn about different types of sex toys and other pleasure-enhancing products in a way that feels approachable, fun, and light-hearted.

At a sex toy party, you'll typically join a small group of friends or acquaintances in someone's home or a private location. The atmosphere is relaxed, and the focus is on education and exploration. A knowledgeable consultant leads the event, showcasing various products such as vibrators, lubricants, massage oils, and other intimate items. You'll have the chance to ask questions, handle the products, and purchase items discreetly if something piques your interest.

What makes these parties appealing is that they provide an opportunity to talk openly about sex and pleasure in a supportive and non-judgmental environment. For many older adults, it's a chance to explore a side of their sexuality they may not have given much thought to in years. Plus, the social aspect can make the experience more enjoyable and less intimidating.

Sex toy parties aren't just about buying products—they're about empowerment and education. Whether you're single or in a relationship, these events can help you learn more about your body, discover new ways to experience pleasure, and feel more comfortable discussing your sexual health.

Case History: Martha's Celebration of Health

Martha, a recent transplant to The Villages from Boston, brought with her not only her distinct accent but a fresh perspective on sexual wellness. After attending a sex toy party hosted by an old college friend back in Boston, she was inspired to introduce a similar concept to her new community. With her signature enthusiasm, Martha hosted a "pleasure party," inviting her closest friends into her beautifully decorated home.

The event featured a variety of sex toys, lubricants, and educational materials, with a professional consultant on hand to explain the benefits of each product. There was a mix of curiosity and apprehension when her guests first arrived. However, Martha's welcoming nature quickly eased the atmosphere. The consultant led an engaging discussion on sexual health as we age, explaining how these products could enhance both personal satisfaction and intimacy with a partner.

What began as a cautious gathering soon became an evening filled with laughter, lively discussions, and genuine curiosity. As questions flowed and conversations deepened, Martha's friends became more open to the idea of exploring new ways to prioritize their sexual wellness. By the end of the night, the group left feeling empowered and inspired, grateful for the opportunity to discuss and embrace this often-overlooked part of life.

Martha's initiative demonstrated that it's never too late to explore new experiences. Her event fostered meaningful conversations about intimacy and also strengthened friendships within her community, proving that staying curious and open-minded can enhance individual well-being and collective connection.

Key Lessons:

- **Deepen Intimacy and Pleasure:** The consultant shared how sex toys can bring new sensations and variety into a relationship, keeping things fresh and exciting. Martha's friends were especially interested in how some vibrators could help with common age-related issues like decreased arousal or dryness, opening up new possibilities for connection and pleasure.

- **Promote Sexual Health and Wellness:** The consultant shared how sex toys can bring new sensations and variety into a relationship, keeping things fresh and exciting. Martha's friends were especially interested in how some vibrators could help with common age-related issues like decreased arousal or dryness, opening up new possibilities for connection and pleasure.

- **Encourage Honest Communication:** Martha's event created a relaxed and open environment where her friends could explore their curiosities without feeling judged. This sense of comfort made sex toys less intimidating and enabled more open discussions about their sexual needs and desires. As a result, attendees felt empowered to communicate more openly with their partners and take control of their sexual well-being.

Sex Toys Made Simple

Sex toys are specifically designed to provide comfort and pleasure, even if you face challenges like limited mobility or reduced sensation. The secret lies in selecting toys that are easy to use, with ergonomic designs that fit comfortably in your hand and are simple to control. Here are some of the best sex toys for older adults that can enhance your intimate experiences and help you rediscover pleasure.

Sex toys can enhance sexual pleasure for older adults, helping to overcome physical limitations

Ergonomically Designed Vibrators

Vibrators are crafted with user-friendly handles and ergonomic shapes, designed to fit naturally and comfortably in your hand. These features ensure the toy is easy to use and enhances your overall experience. For individuals dealing with arthritis or limited hand mobility, these ergonomic designs are particularly beneficial. They reduce the strain on your joints and muscles, making them easier to hold and operate for longer periods without discomfort.

Dual-Stimulation Vibrators

Dual-stimulation vibrators are designed to deliver pleasure both internally and externally at the same time. These well-crafted toys stimulate multiple erogenous zones, offering a more complete and satisfying experience. For those with reduced sensitivity, the dual-action function can be beneficial, as it intensifies sensations and enhances overall enjoyment.

Rechargeable Wand Massagers

Rechargeable wand massagers are powerful tools designed to elevate your pleasure. With a range of vibration settings and rechargeable batteries, they offer both versatility and convenience. The benefit of rechargeable batteries means you won't have to worry about the hassle of replacing batteries or losing power in the middle of your experience. This combination of strength and ease of use ensures you can enjoy continuous, uninterrupted pleasure, making them a great option for a reliable and satisfying experience.

Remote-Controlled Devices

Remote-controlled devices introduce a new level of innovation to your intimate moments. Operable via a remote control or a smartphone app, these toys offer the convenience of hands-free control. This means you can adjust settings and intensities without interrupting your experience, allowing for playful interaction and spontaneity. The remote or app-based control frees you from manual adjustments, making it easier to explore new sensations and enjoy intimacy in a fun and dynamic way.

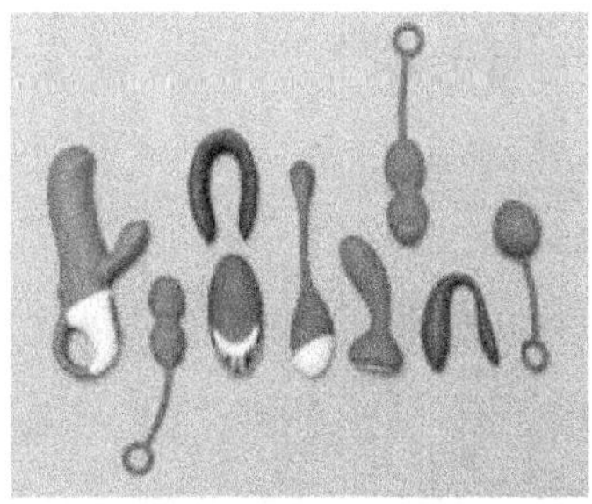

Penis Rings

Penis rings are worn around the base of the penis to help sustain firmer, longer-lasting erections by gently restricting blood flow. This added support can provide more control over erections, making them stronger and more enduring. If you're dealing with erectile dysfunction (ED), penis rings offer a simple and effective way to enhance sexual performance. Using one can improve your intimate experiences and boost your confidence.

G-Spot Stimulators

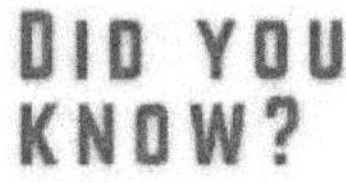
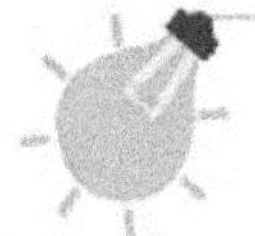

G-spot stimulators are crafted to provide precise and targeted stimulation to the G-spot, offering a pathway to intense pleasure. These expertly designed toys are tailored to reach and effectively stimulate this sensitive area, ensuring maximum satisfaction. Their ergonomic shape makes them easy to position and use, enhancing comfort and enjoyment during intimate moments. G-spot stimulators allow you to experience more profound and fulfilling sensations by focusing on this erogenous zone.

Clitoral Suction Devices

Clitoral suction devices are designed to bring unparalleled pleasure by stimulating the clitoris with gentle, rhythmic suction. These intimate toys create a unique sensation that closely mimics the feeling of oral stimulation, providing a deeply satisfying and intensely pleasurable experience. If you have reduced clitoral sensitivity, these devices can be especially useful, as they offer focused and effective stimulation. The gentle suction enhances sensitivity, leading to more intense and satisfying orgasms. Their targeted approach ensures you enjoy an intensely pleasurable experience, perfectly catering to your needs and preferences.

Flexible Dildos

Flexible dildos are crafted from body-safe materials and designed to bend and adapt to various angles and positions, ensuring a personalized and pleasurable experience. Their flexibility allows you to explore different movements and sensations, providing maximum comfort and satisfaction. These dildos cater to your unique body shape and preferences, making finding the most enjoyable positions easier. Their ability to bend and adjust means you can discover new ways to enhance your intimate moments.

Lube It Up!

While lubricants aren't sex toys, they are essential for enhancing your experience with them, ensuring more comfortable and pleasurable intimate moments. Personal lubricants come in various types, from water-based to silicone-based options, ensuring you can find the perfect match for your needs. Whether you're new to using lubricants or just looking for useful tips, you'll discover valuable insights to enhance your experience. Let's dive into the different types of lubricants and how they can increase your comfort, making intimate moments smoother and more pleasurable.

Water-Based Lubricants

Water-based lubricants are a popular, versatile choice that's easy to use and widely compatible. Since they're made mostly from water, these lubricants come in different textures, from light and silky to thick and gel-like, allowing you to choose the consistency that suits your preferences. They provide smooth, friction-free lubrication, enhancing comfort and pleasure. Safe to use with all types of condoms and sex toys, you won't have to worry about damaging your favorite products. Cleanup is simple and mess-free, as they leave no stains behind. Plus, with hypoallergenic options, even those with sensitive skin can enjoy these lubricants without irritation.

Silicone-Based Lubricants

Silicone-based lubricants provide a silky, luxurious feel, making them perfect for longer-lasting pleasure. Unlike water-based lubricants, they don't dry out quickly, so you can enjoy a smooth and indulgent experience without needing to reapply often. Waterproof and hypoallergenic, these lubricants are ideal for sensitive skin and are perfect for use in the shower or bath. Silicone-based lubricants shouldn't be used with silicone sex toys, as they can chemically react with the material, potentially causing damage and encouraging bacterial growth.

Oil-Based Lubricants

Oil-based lubricants, made from natural oils like coconut or olive oil, offer a thick, soothing glide that enhances intimacy and lasts longer than water-based alternatives. These lubricants provide a rich, moisturizing feel, reducing the need for frequent reapplication. However, it's important to note that oil-based lubricants aren't safe to use with latex condoms, as they can weaken the material and reduce its effectiveness. They may also be more difficult to clean from skin and fabrics and, in some cases, can clog pores or cause irritation. While oil-based lubricants can be an excellent option for long-lasting pleasure, they're best suited for situations where condoms aren't needed and when you're seeking a deeply moisturizing, extended experience.

Hybrid Lubricants (Water and Silicone Mix)

Hybrid lubricants combine the best of both worlds—the ease and comfort of water-based formulas with the long-lasting smoothness of silicone. These innovative blends offer a silky, balanced glide that's both practical and pleasurable. With hybrid lubricants, you get the extended endurance of silicone while still enjoying the easy cleanup of a water-based option. They're versatile, compatible with condoms and most toys, and provide a luxurious, long-lasting experience, making them perfect for any intimate occasion.

Natural and Organic Lubricants

Natural and organic lubricants provide a gentle, eco-friendly choice for intimate moments. Made from pure, biodegradable ingredients, they are perfect for those with sensitive skin or who prioritize a clean, green lifestyle. Free from parabens, glycerin, and synthetic fragrances, these lubricants reduce the risk of irritation while offering a soothing, natural experience. Choosing natural and organic lubricants allows you to enjoy intimacy with confidence, knowing you're using a product that's not only kind to your body but also to the planet.

Flavored and Sensation Lubricants

Enhance your intimate moments with flavored and sensation lubricants that add a playful, exciting touch. Whether savoring a delicious flavor or indulging in a warming or cooling sensation, these lubricants are designed to amplify pleasure and bring a new level of fun to your encounters. Flavored options make oral sex more enjoyable while warming or cooling effects create a thrilling, unexpected twist. With a wide range of flavors and sensations, you can easily find the perfect lubricant to spice up your experience and keep things fresh and exciting.

Tips:

- **Choose the Right Sex Toy:** Select toys with ergonomic designs that minimize strain and enhance comfort. Look for toys with adjustable settings so you can control the intensity and speed to match your preferences. Beginners may prefer smaller, straightforward designs, while more advanced users might enjoy more intricate or larger options. Prioritize toys made from safe materials, like medical-grade silicone, which are non-toxic and easy to clean. Waterproof toys are a great option for ease of cleaning and versatility in use.

- **Pick the Right Lubricant:** Choose lubricants made for mature skin, focusing on formulas that hydrate and soothe. Look for ingredients like aloe vera or hyaluronic acid to help combat dryness and provide a smoother experience. Select hypoallergenic lubricants free from irritants like glycerin, parabens, and fragrances for greater comfort and satisfaction.

CHAPTER 15

Switch It Up!

"Don't be afraid to experiment. Everything new is an opportunity for pleasure."

— Mae West, American Actress

Exploring Sexual Positions

As we journey through life, our bodies and needs evolve, and so too does our approach to intimacy. For older adults, maintaining a fulfilling and pleasurable sexual connection is not only possible but can deepen with age. However, changes in flexibility, joint health, stamina, and other factors can influence how we experience physical intimacy. These natural changes present an opportunity to explore new ways to engage with your partner through creative adjustments in sexual positions, ensuring comfort and satisfaction.

Sexual expression in later life is about more than just the physical act—it's about connection, communication, and the shared desire to maintain intimacy. While certain positions that were once comfortable may need modification, this chapter is designed to guide you through options that are not only pleasurable but also practical. Each position discussed is adaptable, offering variations that take into account physical limitations while enhancing the emotional connection between you and your partner. Exploring sexual positions is a way to enhance intimacy and also prioritize comfort, adaptability, and respect for our body's unique limits. Whether you're navigating arthritis, limited flexibility, or simply looking to connect in fresh ways, these options provide pathways to deepen connection and enjoyment with minimal physical strain.

New Adventures, New Pleasures

Here are some leading sexual positions that take into account the unique physical changes and abilities that come with aging. These positions are designed to enhance pleasure while ensuring that you and your partner feel comfortable and connected.

Spoon Position

Description: Both partners lie on their sides facing the same direction—the receiving partner curls into a fetal position while the penetrating partner aligns their hips behind for penetration.

Benefits: This position reduces strain on joints and muscles, making it particularly suitable for individuals with arthritis or mobility issues. Additionally, this position's close, comforting body contact promotes a sense of intimacy between partners.

Seated Edge Position

Description: The receiving partner sits on the edge of a sturdy chair or bed while the penetrating partner stands or kneels in front. The receiving partner can lean back for support.

Benefits: This position allows for deep penetration with minimal strain, ensuring comfort and ease. The support provided by the chair or bed reduces the risk of discomfort, making it an accessible option for various physical conditions and preferences.

Woman on Top (Cowgirl)

Description: The penetrating partner lies on their back while the receiving partner straddles them, facing forward.

Benefits: This position gives control to the receiving partner, allowing them to adjust the angle and speed to their comfort and preference. It reduces lower back strain for the penetrating partner and offers a variety of angles and sensations for both partners.

Reverse Cowgirl

Description: The penetrating partner lies on their back, and the receiving partner straddles them while facing away.

Benefits: This position controls the receiving partner, allowing them to dictate the pace and depth of penetration according to their comfort. It reduces pressure on the knees, making it easier to maintain for extended periods. Additionally, it offers a different angle of penetration, which can enhance stimulation and pleasure.

Face-to-Face Sitting Position

Description: Both partners sit facing each other on a bed or a sturdy chair, with legs wrapped around each other.

Benefits: This position significantly enhances intimacy by allowing partners to maintain eye contact and close physical connection. It provides mutual support, as both partners can lean on each other for stability. Additionally, it helps manage balance, making it a comfortable and secure option for various physical abilities.

Side-by-Side (Side-Lying)

Description: Both partners lie on their sides facing each other, with the penetrating partner lifting the receiving partner's leg for penetration.

Benefits: This position is gentle on the joints, making it suitable for those with mobility issues. It allows for close physical contact and accessible communication, enabling partners to make adjustments comfortably and ensuring a mutually satisfying experience.

Modified Missionary

Description: The receiving partner lies on their back with a pillow under their hips, and the penetrating partner kneels or stands at the edge of the bed.

Benefits: This position reduces strain on the back and knees, making it more comfortable for both partners. It allows for eye contact, which can enhance intimacy and emotional connection. Additionally, the pillow supports the receiving partner's hips, helping to achieve a more comfortable and practical angle for penetration.

Butterfly Position

Description: The receiving partner lies on their back at the edge of the bed with their legs spread while the penetrating partner stands or kneels between their legs.

Benefits: This position supports both partners, allowing the receiving partner to rest comfortably on the bed. It enables deep penetration, enhancing physical connection and pleasure. It also reduces strain on the back and knees, making it more sustainable and comfortable for longer durations.

Lotus Position

Description: The penetrating partner sits cross-legged, and the receiving partner sits on their lap facing them, wrapping their legs around the penetrating partner's waist.

Benefits: This position enhances intimacy and emotional connection by allowing partners to maintain close eye contact and physical proximity. It allows for slow and controlled movement, which can be incredibly pleasurable and comfortable. Additionally, it provides mutual support, as both partners can rely on each other for stability and balance.

Standing Supported

Description: The receiving partner stands with their back against a wall for support, and the penetrating partner stands facing them, lifting one of the receiving partner's legs.

Benefits: This position provides sturdy wall support, helping maintain balance and stability. It reduces strain on the back, making it more comfortable for both partners. Additionally, it allows for varied angles and penetration depths, enhancing versatility and pleasure.

Tips:

- **Prioritize Comfort:** Choose positions that reduce strain on your joints and muscles. Use pillows, cushions, or wedges to support your body and make the experience more relaxing and enjoyable.

- **Communicate Openly:** Honest conversations with your partner about your sexual preferences and needs are crucial. Open dialogue ensures you feel comfortable, respected, and able to explore positions that work best for your body.

- **Take Your Time:** Go slowly when trying out new positions. Moving gently allows your body to adjust without discomfort and can enhance your experience together.

- **Modify Traditional Positions:** Don't hesitate to adapt classic positions to suit your physical needs. For instance, side-lying positions can ease pressure on sensitive areas like your knees or back, making them more comfortable for longer periods.

- **Use Your Environment:** Incorporating sturdy furniture into your intimate experiences can provide extra support. A chair, firm mattress, or countertop can offer stability, reducing strain on your body.

- **Stay Flexible:** Gentle stretching exercises in your daily routine can enhance your flexibility, which will help you feel more comfortable trying new sexual positions. Daily movement can go a long way in enhancing your physical readiness.

- **Lubrication is Essential:** As natural lubrication tends to decrease with age, a high-quality lubricant can greatly enhance comfort and make intimate moments more pleasurable. Keep it handy to ensure smooth and enjoyable experiences.

- **Stay Curious:** Don't hesitate to explore resources specifically tailored to older adults. Books, guides, or instructional videos can provide ideas for comfortable and satisfying positions.

CHAPTER 16

Virtual Sex Apps

"The future of sex is digital, where AI will learn our desires and fulfill them in ways we haven't yet imagined."

— Kate Devlin, British Author

Sex and AI: A New Era

The future of sexual health and aging is filled with promise and potential. With breakthroughs in medical research, cutting-edge technology, and an increased focus on education, there are more ways than ever for you to nurture and enhance your sexual well-being. These advancements are leading to more innovative approaches to sexual health for older adults, helping you maintain intimacy and satisfaction throughout your life.

A particularly exciting development in this realm is the use of artificial intelligence (AI) in healthcare, including sexual health. AI is revolutionizing healthcare delivery by analyzing vast amounts of data, providing personalized treatments, and engaging with patients in new and dynamic ways. Here's how AI is shaping the future of sexual health.

Data Analysis

AI's ability to process large datasets allows for identifying patterns and trends that traditional methods may miss. This leads to more accurate diagnoses of sexual health issues such as erectile dysfunction (ED), hormonal imbalances, and STIs—enabling quicker and more effective treatment.

Personalized Treatments

AI can analyze your medical history, lifestyle choices, and genetic makeup to identify and predict sexual health issues before they develop. This forward-thinking method enables early detection and creates customized treatment plans tailored to your unique needs, ensuring you can address issues promptly and maintain a vibrant and satisfying intimate life.

AI Platforms, Apps, and Chatbots

AI platforms like IBM Watson Health can measure your health conditions and the medications you are taking to provide safe and effective care. These systems can monitor your health in real-time, adjusting treatments to match your needs. This personalized approach makes managing your sexual health more accessible and practical.

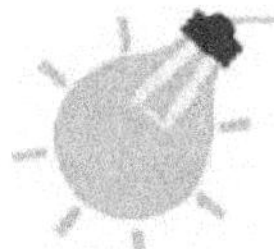

AI-driven apps offer easy-to-use educational modules on sexuality. These tools offer expert knowledge and practical learning directly to your device, helping you stay informed and take control of your sexual health. You can learn about safe sex practices, STI prevention, and managing sexual dysfunction. The AI in the app will give you personalized recommendations for further reading, exercises, or consultations with healthcare professionals. This makes learning about sexual health simple, engaging, and effective.

AI-driven chatbots and virtual health assistants (VHAs) are accessible 24/7, ready to answer questions about your health, medications, and treatment options. This can be particularly useful for individuals with mobility challenges or those living in remote areas. For many, discussing sexual health face-to-face can feel uncomfortable. These technologies provide a more discreet and private way to get the information you need, helping to reduce stigma and allowing you to address sexual health concerns with greater comfort and confidence.

Wearable Tech

Wearable technology is changing how you care for your health by providing continuous, real-time monitoring. Devices like fitness trackers and smartwatches make it easy to keep track of important health markers such as heart rate, blood pressure, sleep quality, and stress levels. They can also remind you to take your medications and follow your treatment plans. These tools act like personal health assistants, providing constant insight into your well-being.

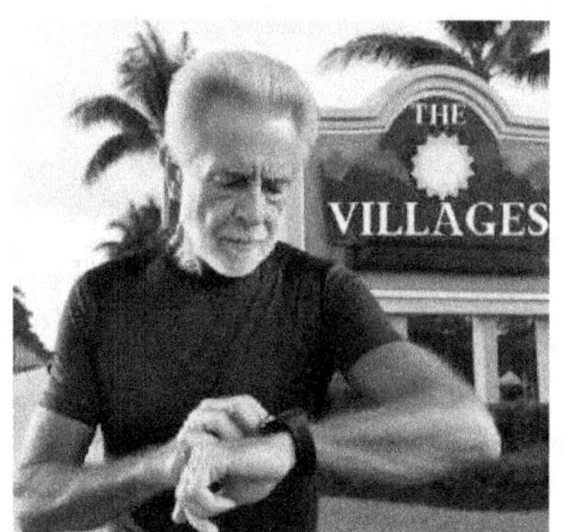

One important feature of these devices is their ability to measure heart rate variability (HRV), which is the time difference between heartbeats. A higher HRV generally means your heart is healthier and better able to handle stress.

Your sleep patterns can also be tracked, helping you understand how well you're resting. Getting good sleep is key to reducing stress, balancing hormones, and keeping your energy levels up—all of which contribute to maintaining a fulfilling, intimate life.

Beyond physical health, wearable devices can also support your mental well-being. They monitor stress, mood, and anxiety levels, offering real-time feedback. This can help you manage stress by encouraging relaxation techniques like mindfulness or deep breathing. Lowering stress improves your mental well-being and helps you build stronger emotional connections. It also eases performance anxiety, which can lead to a more fulfilling and satisfying sexual experience.

AR and VR to Enhance Sexuality

As technology advances, innovative tools like augmented reality (AR) and virtual reality (VR) are becoming more available, offering exciting new ways to enhance daily life. These cutting-edge technologies open up fresh possibilities to improve sexual health and intimacy by addressing the challenges that often arise with aging. To understand their potential, let's explore what AR and VR are, how they function, and how they can positively impact your sexual wellness.

What is Augmented Reality (AR)?

Augmented reality (AR) adds a digital layer to the world around you, blending virtual elements like images, sounds, or information with what you see in real life. It enhances your surroundings without taking you out of them. A simple example is using your phone to see how furniture would look in your home before buying it. Apps like IKEA let you point your camera at your living room and place a digital version of a chair or table right in the space, helping you easily make decisions.

AR and Sexual Health for Older Adults

- **Building Intimacy:** AR can help strengthen emotional connections between partners by providing interactive activities that promote bonding. Whether it's exploring new ways to communicate or enjoying shared virtual experiences, AR allows you to engage with your partner in fun, meaningful ways that can deepen your relationship and enhance intimacy.

- **Sex Education:** AR can offer a personalized approach to learning about sexual health, making information easier to understand and apply. You can access interactive guides that explain age-related changes, safe practices, and ways to improve your sexual well-being—all in a way that feels approachable and tailored to your needs.

- **Enhanced Sensory Experience:** With AR, you can enjoy enriched sensory experiences that stimulate your mind and body. These virtual enhancements can be beneficial in overcoming physical limitations that may come with aging, allowing you to explore new dimensions of pleasure and connection in a safe, comfortable environment.

What is Virtual Reality (VR)?

Virtual reality (VR) immerses you in a completely digital world, allowing you to experience and interact with virtual surroundings as if they were real. When you wear a VR headset, you're transported into a new environment where you can see, hear, and sometimes even feel the virtual objects around you. Unlike Augmented Reality, which enhances your real-world view, VR creates an entirely different space. For instance, you can take virtual tours of famous places like museums, cities, or natural wonders. Imagine exploring the Louvre Museum in Paris without ever leaving your home.

VR and Sexual Health for Older Adults

- **Creating Romantic Experiences:** VR can help you and your partner create unforgettable romantic moments, even from a distance. Whether sharing a virtual sunset on a beach or exploring a dream destination together, VR offers a way to connect intimately through shared experiences. These digital adventures can reignite passion and build closeness no matter where you are.

- **Sexual Health Therapy:** VR provides a safe and controlled environment for therapeutic interventions related to sexual health. It can assist in addressing common age-related issues like performance anxiety, sexual dysfunction, or body image concerns. Through immersive programs, you can explore techniques to improve sexual wellness, practice relaxation exercises, and learn strategies for overcoming specific challenges—all at your own pace and comfort.

- **Stimulating New Experiences:** VR transports you into vivid, realistic environments that fully engage your senses, allowing you to experience connection and pleasure in new, exciting ways. Even if you face physical limitations, VR provides a unique opportunity to explore intimacy and enjoyment by creating immersive experiences that feel real, helping you reconnect with sensations and emotions that enhance your overall well-being. This technology empowers you to rediscover joy and fulfillment in a comfortable, accessible manner, opening doors to excitement and satisfaction that may have once felt out of reach.

Augmented reality (AR) and virtual reality (VR) are revolutionizing how we experience the world. These innovative technologies provide new, engaging ways to support and enhance your sexual health and intimacy. By embracing AR and VR, you can enjoy immersive experiences that enable deeper connections and more satisfying relationships. Regardless of your age or physical challenges, these tools offer exciting possibilities to maintain and even improve your sexual wellness, helping you experience a richer, more fulfilling sense of connection.

Tips:

- **Discover AR and VR for Sexual Wellness:** Virtual reality (VR) and augmented reality (AR) open the door to new and exciting ways to explore your sexual health. Don't hesitate to try something different. Experiment with these tools to enhance intimacy, explore fantasies, and create enjoyable experiences in a safe and comfortable environment.

- **Enhance Connection and Wellness:** Whether you're in a relationship or on your own, AR and VR can help you build deeper emotional connections and improve your sense of well-being. If you have a partner, use these technologies to create shared experiences that bring you closer. If you're solo, explore ways to boost personal fulfillment and wellness through immersive virtual environments.

CHAPTER 17
Robo-Relations

"Sex with robots could lead to the perfect, custom-designed partner, one that could never exist in real life."
— Janna Levin, American Author and Astronomer

Companion Robots

Remember the futuristic world of *The Jetsons* and their helpful robot, Rosie? What once seemed like science fiction is now becoming a reality. Technology has come a long way, and companion robots are no longer just a cartoon fantasy. Today, these advanced robots are here to offer real assistance, emotional support, and companionship—helping you live more independently.

Emotional, Cognitive, and Social Support

Companion robots can brighten your day by providing conversation and emotional comfort, especially if you're living alone. Many older adults experience feelings of loneliness and isolation, which can negatively impact emotional health. Companion robots provide consistent companionship, easing loneliness through regular interaction, conversation, and playful engagement. These robots will become a source of emotional comfort, helping to reduce stress and elevate mood.

In addition to emotional support, companion robots play a crucial role in maintaining cognitive health. They can participate in interactive games, puzzles, and other stimulating activities, challenge memory, enhance problem-solving skills, and boost critical thinking. This cognitive engagement keeps your brain active and sharp, helping to slow the natural progression of mental decline that can occur with aging.

Moreover, companion robots can act as social facilitators, connecting you with friends and family. They can make video calls, send messages, and remind you of important dates and events, ensuring you stay socially engaged and connected. Companion robots can play a vital role in supporting your overall well-being through emotional support, mental stimulation, and maintaining social connections.

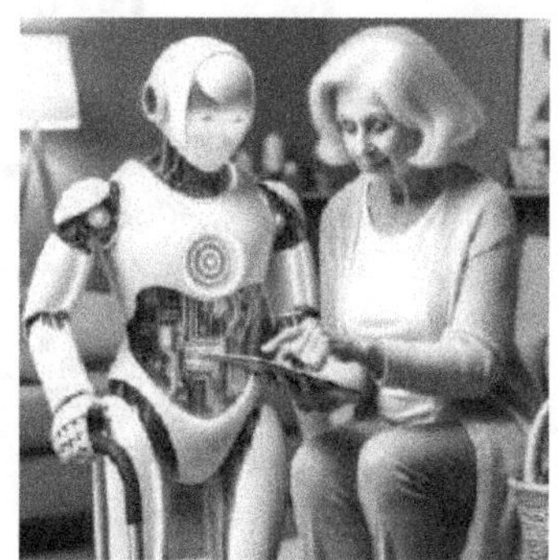

Assisting with Daily Tasks

Beyond companionship, companion robots offer invaluable support in managing daily tasks—whether it's reminding you to take your medications, preparing meals, managing household chores, or even helping you stay organized. By providing gentle reminders and assistance, companion robots allow you to focus on what matters most while ensuring your daily routine stays on track. These robots are designed to improve your quality of life, keeping you active and engaged while offering a sense of freedom and independence that you can rely on.

Supporting Healthy Habits

Companion robots can play a key role in helping you establish and maintain healthy habits by providing timely reminders and encouragement. Whether it's prompting you to engage in regular physical activity or follow a balanced diet, these robots serve as personalized wellness coaches. They can also track your progress, offering gentle nudges to stay on course with your health goals.

Health Monitoring

These robots come equipped with advanced health monitoring features, transforming how we manage our well-being. Companion robots will track vital health metrics such as heart rate, blood pressure, sleep patterns, and physical activity, providing real-time data that can help detect potential health issues early. In addition to tracking, they will remind you of medical appointments, assist with medication schedules, and even alert healthcare providers in emergencies or when intervention is needed.

Enhancing Safety and Security

Safety becomes even more important as you age, especially if you live alone. Companion robots offer a practical solution by adding an extra layer of security to your daily life. These robots are designed to monitor your home and can alert caregivers or emergency services when needed. For example, if you experience a fall, your robot can instantly detect it and call for help, ensuring you're never left alone in an emergency.

In addition to emergency support, companion robots provide helpful reminders to keep you safe, such as locking doors and turning off appliances. With these safety measures in place, you can feel more secure and confident in your ability to live independently.

Future of Companion Robots

Companion robots are rapidly becoming common in homes, especially among older adults and those seeking additional support for daily living. Soon, their integration into households will become even more widespread, enhancing independence and improving quality of life. As people grow more familiar with their capabilities, companion robots will play an increasingly vital role in promoting well-being and maintaining social connections.

Advanced Emotional Interaction

Imagine a future where companion robots bring a new level of emotional intelligence into your life. These robots won't just talk to you—they'll engage in rich conversations, recognizing familiar faces and responding to your unique moods. With the ability to interpret your emotions, they'll offer comfort, support, and companionship in a way that feels remarkably human. As they learn from your routines, preferences, and past interactions, these robots will adapt, offering personalized care and assistance that aligns perfectly with your needs. Over time, they'll become more intuitive, providing health insights, reminders, and tailored support—creating interactions that feel increasingly natural and meaningful.

Customized Companionship

Imagine a companion robot that truly understands you. These future robots will get to know your personality, habits, and even quirks—becoming a partner in your favorite hobbies, sparking conversations on topics you love, or introducing you to new activities that fit your style. Every interaction will feel natural and enjoyable as the robot aligns itself with your evolving interests and needs, making the companionship genuinely fulfilling.

Physical Empowerment

Tomorrow's robots will offer much more than simple assistance; they'll empower you physically. Whether guiding you through exercises, helping with mobility, or assisting with personal care, they'll adapt to your physical needs to keep you feeling capable and energetic. This added support can boost your well-being and confidence, helping you feel at ease and comfortable in every aspect of your life.

Case History: Samantha's High-Tech Romance

In The Villages, where sunshine and socializing fill every corner, lived Samantha—a savvy retiree with deep family roots in real estate. One sunny afternoon, she struck up a conversation at the newly developed Lake Sumter

Landing. Samantha's excitement was contagious as she shared her latest passion for tech. "I'm mastering my new smartphone!" she laughed, her eyes alight with curiosity. She was on a journey, eager to dive into the world of digital innovation and the unexpected ways it could enrich her life.

"These are my golden years, and I'm determined to make them sparkle," she declared. Her mission went far beyond basic gadgets—she explored apps, devices, and even digital tools to elevate her health and enhance her lifestyle. "Can you believe all these wellness apps? There's even a dating app for people like us!" she giggled. With a playful grin, she added, "You know, a robot companion would be perfect for me. I'd call him Romeo—he'd never argue or hog the remote!"

As her fascination deepened, Samantha uncovered gadgets she'd never dreamed of. One of her favorites was a wearable that tracked her hormones, which she lovingly referred to as her "libido coach." With humor intact, she faced challenges, like mastering a smart pelvic floor trainer. "Who knew staying healthy required so much reading?" she joked, unfazed by the technical hurdles.

Samantha's tech journey soon inspired her friends to join in. Encouraged by her zeal, they traded their old phones for smartphones and joined fitness apps to keep tabs on each other's progress. What began as a quirky hobby became a community effort, with everyone cheering each other on. "I may be single, but I've got a whole team now!" she laughed.

In embracing the world of tech, Samantha discovered something deeper—an evolving sense of herself. "This isn't just about learning gadgets; it's about rediscovering who I am," she reflected. Her resilience and wit made her a beloved figure in The Villages. "I've got wonderful friends, and who knows? Maybe a future with Romeo," she teased, fully aware of the pioneering spirit she embodied. Though Samantha didn't live to see companion robots become mainstream, her adventurous spirit was a sign of things to come— proving that age is no barrier to curiosity and reinvention.

Key Lessons:

- **Keep an Open Mind and Embrace the Unknown**: Samantha's enthusiasm for technology reminds us that curiosity can lead to wonderful surprises. Whether experimenting with new gadgets or diving into something unfamiliar, staying open-minded can reveal new insights about yourself and add excitement to your journey.

- **Tackle Challenges with a Smile**: Samantha's upbeat approach to navigating tricky gadgets shows the impact of a positive outlook. Facing obstacles with humor and resilience makes them more bearable and can turn them into memorable, even fun, experiences.

- **Make Self-Care a Priority**: Samantha's journey highlights the importance of nurturing your well-being. She shows that self-care is a lifelong investment by focusing on self-discovery and exploring tools to support her health. Taking care of yourself at every age helps you keep growing and thriving.

Sex Robots

As technology continues to change our world, many new inventions offer unique ways to enhance companionship, connection, and intimacy. One such innovation is the sex robot—a new device designed to look, feel, and interact like a real partner. For some, the idea of a robot providing companionship and physical connection may seem futuristic, even a little strange. But as our society evolves, so do our options for creating comfort, pleasure, and support at every stage of life.

Sex robots are more than just machines. They are highly advanced, interactive robots designed to respond to touch, voice, and other inputs, offering companionship and intimacy in a way that many people find fulfilling. These robots are designed to be lifelike, with soft skin, realistic features, and sometimes even personalities. They can converse, remember your preferences, and respond to your needs, making them much more than a typical gadget.

Safe Outlet for Sexual Expression

As we get older, society's views on sexual expression can sometimes feel dismissive or even judgmental, creating unnecessary barriers to exploring and

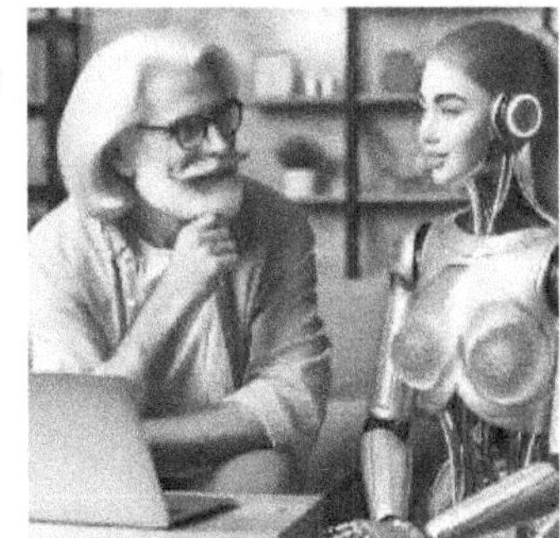

enjoying this natural part of life. Sex robots provide a private, stigma-free way to experience intimacy on your own terms, allowing you to express your desires without the worry of outside judgment or societal pressures.

In many retirement communities, discussions around safe sex practices are often limited, which can unfortunately lead to a higher risk of sexually transmitted infections (STIs). Sex robots offer a safe and worry-free alternative, allowing you to engage in intimate experiences while reducing exposure to these health risks. This new option not only supports a healthier approach to sexual wellness but also empowers you to explore intimacy confidently, safely, and without compromise.

Future of Sex Robots

Sex robots are becoming more accessible and will likely gain greater social acceptance as they evolve. With technological advancements, these robots will offer increasingly sophisticated interactions, combining physical realism with advanced artificial intelligence.

Personalized Experiences

In the future, sex robots will offer an unmatched level of customization, allowing you to choose everything from facial features and body type to skin tone, hair, and eye color. You'll be able to personalize the robot's appearance and personality, with options to select traits like shy, intellectual, sensual, or adventurous—all through an easy-to-use mobile app. As you interact, these robots will learn your unique preferences and desires, adapting to your tastes and making each experience feel increasingly personal and fulfilling.

These future models will move and respond in lifelike ways, with advanced sensors that detect and respond to touch, making your interactions feel natural and engaging. As technology continues to evolve, sex robots could play a larger role in how people explore companionship, connection, and well-being. With the ability to adapt to your needs, they will offer a private, judgment-free space to explore intimacy in ways that suit you. The rise of sex robots will also shape societal perspectives on relationships and sexual health, opening new pathways for connection and satisfaction.

Considerations Before Buying a Robot

While companion and sex robots bring exciting possibilities for connection and support, they also raise important ethical, social, and legal questions worth considering.

Ethical Love

One consideration is the potential for becoming emotionally dependent on a robot, which could impact how you relate to others. With highly responsive and interactive features, these robots can feel deeply engaging, but this reliance may unintentionally lead to social withdrawal or even reshape your expectations of human relationships. Balancing these experiences with genuine human interaction is essential to keep relationships fulfilling and authentic.

Privacy and Data Security

Many robots rely on personal information to tailor their responses and actions, raising concerns about privacy and security. Sensitive data, from personal preferences to biometric information, could be at risk without stringent protections. Before purchasing, it's wise to research the manufacturer's approach to data privacy, ensuring safeguards are in place to prevent unauthorized access or misuse of your personal information.

Equity in Access

As with many advanced technologies, cost and accessibility are major factors. If robots remain costly, they could be out of reach for many people, potentially widening gaps in access to these forms of companionship and support. Widespread availability and affordability of companion robots will be essential to ensure these benefits are accessible to all, regardless of financial background.

Legal Boundaries

It's also important to be aware of legal guidelines. While adult sex robots and companion robots are generally legal in the U.S. and many other places, there are restrictions in some jurisdictions, especially around products resembling minors. Staying informed on local laws ensures you enjoy your experience responsibly and in compliance with regulations.

Tips:

- **Embrace Emotional Wellness with a Companion Robot:** Invite a companion robot like Moxie (yes, it's available) into your life to enrich emotional wellness and reduce isolation. With Moxie around, you're gaining a personalized companion who can engage in conversation, provide gentle reminders, and even play music or tell stories. Engaging with Moxie can boost your mood, help you relax, and create a sense of warmth and connection in your home.

- **Consider Exploring Intimacy with a Sex Robot:** If you're ready to rediscover or continue exploring intimacy in a safe, customized way, a sex robot can provide an exciting solution. A sex robot can be designed to cater to your needs, with customizable features that make the experience personal and comfortable. Physical changes can impact intimacy with age, but with a sex robot, you're in control of the experience. A sex robot can support your emotional and physical wellness in ways that can make you feel vibrant, fulfilled, and confident in your sexuality.

CHAPTER 18

The Future is Now!

"The future of sex will be shaped by technology, just as much as it has been by biology."

— Helen Fisher, American Anthropologist

Surgical Breakthroughs

Surgical breakthroughs in sexual health are revolutionizing the way we approach sexual health and wellness, offering innovative solutions to enhance and preserve sexual function. These advancements are designed to address a wide range of concerns, from improving reproductive health to treating conditions that impact sexual satisfaction. As research and technology continue to evolve, these cutting-edge procedures hold the potential to transform lives, ensuring that more individuals can enjoy a healthy, fulfilling sex life. Here are some of the most exciting developments that are reshaping the future of sexual health.

Robotic-Assisted Surgery

Robotic-assisted surgery is revolutionizing many medical fields, including sexual health and medicine. This technology provides greater precision, smaller incisions, and faster recovery times. For instance, if you need prostate surgery, advanced robotic techniques can reduce the risk of nerve damage, helping to preserve erectile function. Similarly, robotic-assisted hysterectomy offers a minimally invasive option with shorter recovery times and fewer complications, helping women maintain their sexual function. As robotic-assisted surgery technologies advance, they promise to have even better outcomes for sexual health.

Advanced Genital Reconstruction

Genital reconstruction surgeries are already available for conditions like congenital anomalies, trauma, and gender affirmation. Future improvements in technology will enhance these results. For example, evolving techniques in gender affirmation surgery are expected to yield more natural outcomes and better sensory results for transgender individuals. Advances in microsurgical techniques for clitoral and penile reconstruction will improve sexual function and appearance for people needing reconstruction due to injury or congenital conditions. These innovations aim to enhance both genital functionality and aesthetics.

Stem Cell and Regenerative Medicine

Stem cell therapy and regenerative medicine offer exciting possibilities for treating sexual health issues. For example, stem cell injections will be able to repair and regenerate damaged erectile tissue, providing a long-term solution for ED. Regenerative techniques using stem cells and growth factors will also improve vaginal elasticity, and lubrication, enhancing sexual health and satisfaction.

Pelvic Floor Repair and Reconstruction

Advances in pelvic floor surgery will significantly improve sexual health, especially for adults dealing with age-related issues. Minimally invasive techniques for pelvic organ repair will offer better support and function, leading to improved sexual health outcomes. Enhanced methods for urinary incontinence surgery will also enhance sexual function. These advancements provide practical solutions for maintaining a healthy and satisfying sex life.

Neuromodulation for Sexual Dysfunction

Neuromodulation uses electrical stimulation to alter nerve activity and could offer new treatments for sexual dysfunction. For instance, neuromodulation devices might provide an alternative to medications for ED by directly stimulating the nerves involved in erections. Techniques for stimulating pelvic nerves in females could enhance arousal and improve orgasm. These new treatments have the potential to significantly improve sexual function.

Penile Implants and Prosthetics

Penile implants have been used to treat ED for decades, and future advancements will likely enhance their functionality and comfort. Next-generation implants promise more natural erections, greater control, and improved sensory feedback. Future penile prosthetics will integrate digital technology. This will allow for greater customization and monitoring, leading to enhanced sexual function.

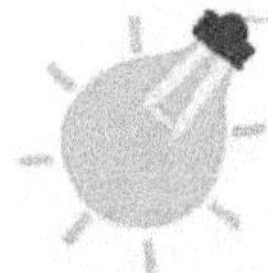

The Future of Sex Tech

The future of sexual health is evolving—and it directly impacts you! Society is finally recognizing that sexual well-being is a lifelong part of health, no matter your age or relationship status. As you navigate your later years, it's important to know that there's growing acceptance of non-traditional relationships, solo intimacy, and the idea that sexual expression changes over time. Technology will transform how you experience intimacy, offering new ways to stay connected, fulfilled, and in touch with your needs.

As innovations in technology continue, they hold the power to revolutionize your sexual health. From personalized health monitoring to AI-driven devices that cater to your preferences, these advancements are designed to help you manage and enhance your sexual well-being. Imagine solutions tailored just for you, ensuring that intimacy and satisfaction remain part of your life. Embrace these changes and allow technology to enrich your relationships and your sense of self as you age—because sexual fulfillment doesn't stop with time; it evolves—just like you do.

Tips:

- **Embrace the Future of Sexual Health:** AI technology is advancing quickly, offering innovative ways to support your sexual health and well-being. From personalized sexual health solutions to interactive tools that adapt to your needs, the future holds exciting possibilities. Staying open to these advancements can help maintain a vibrant, healthy lifestyle as you age.

- **Stay Informed About Sex Tech:** Sexual health is a vital aspect of your overall well-being at every stage of life. With the rise of AI-driven tools, therapies, and innovative resources, there are now countless opportunities to enrich your intimate experiences. By staying up to date on the latest advancements, you can explore new ways to enhance pleasure, intimacy, and connection—while ensuring your sex life evolves to meet your unique needs and desires.

Conclusion

Sex in The Villages is intended to break down the barriers surrounding aging and sexuality, encouraging open and honest conversations on an often-overlooked topic. This book serves as a guide to embracing your sexuality with confidence and vitality, empowering you to maintain a fulfilling and healthy sexual life as you age.

Sexual health is more than just physical satisfaction; it's about connecting on a deeper level, feeling alive, and enthusiastically welcoming every moment. By prioritizing your sexual well-being, you're choosing to celebrate this vital aspect of wellness with authenticity and delight.

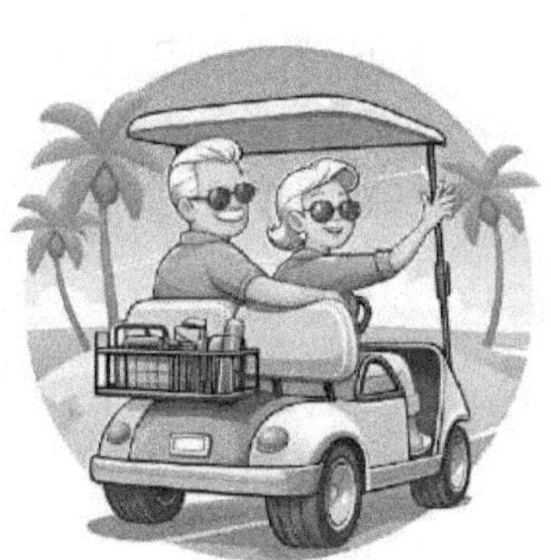

As you close this chapter and embark on your next adventure—whether it's a lively round of golf with friends, a relaxing swim in the pool, or a thoughtful game of chess—remember that aging gracefully involves nurturing every aspect of yourself.

The Villages shows us that life doesn't stop at retirement; it simply shifts into a more relaxed, deeply rewarding phase. By staying active, building strong connections, exploring new hobbies, taking care of your health, approaching relationships with kindness, and finding joy each day—you can enhance your sexual health and overall well-being.

HERE'S TO LIVING—AND LOVING—WELL IN THE VILLAGES!

Thank You!

I want to sincerely thank you for taking the time to read *Sex in The Villages*. I hope you found the information valuable, enlightening, and inspiring for your own journey. If you enjoyed this book or found it helpful, please take a moment to leave a review on the platform where you purchased it. Your feedback helps me improve my work and also assists other readers in discovering this book and the important topics it covers. Thank you again for your time and support!

Warm regards,

Tina M. Penhollow

References

Argiolas, A., Argiolas, F. M., & Argiolas, G., et al. (2023). Erectile dysfunction: Treatments, advances, and new therapeutic strategies. *Brain Sciences, 13*, 802.

Bairstow, A. (2017). Couples exploring nonmonogamy: Guidelines for therapists. *Journal of Sex & Marital Therapy, 43*, 343–353.

Bergstrand, C., & Williams, J. B. (2000). Today's alternative marriage styles: The case of swingers. *Electronic Journal of Human Sexuality*, 3. http://www.ejhs.org/volume3/swing/body.htm.

Bixter, T., Blocker, A., & Rogers, A. (2018). Enhancing social engagement of older adults through technology. *Aging, Technology and Health*, 179-214.

Blanchower, G., & Oswald, J. (2004). Money, sex, and happiness: An empirical study. *Scandinavian Journal of Economics, 106*, 393-415.

Brotto, A., Chivers, L., & Millman, D., et al. (2012). Mindfulness-based sex therapy improves genital-subjective arousal concordance in women with sexual desire/arousal difficulties. *Archives of Sexual Behavior, 41*, 729-740.

Buczak-Stec, E., König, H., & Hajek, A. (2019). The link between sexual satisfaction and subjective well-being: A longitudinal perspective based on the German Ageing Survey. *Quality Life Research, 28*, 3025–3035.

Cameron, J., & Santos-Iglesias, P. (2024). Sexual activity of older adults: A systematic review of the literature. *International Journal of Sexual Health: Official Journal of the World Association for Sexual Health, 36*, 145–166.

Centers for Disease Control and Prevention (CDC). (2024). Sexually transmitted infection rates among adults 55 and older. *AtlasPlus - Charts* (cdc.gov).

Delamater, J., & Koepsel, E. (2015). Relationships and sexual expression in later life: A biopsychosocial perspective. *Sexual and Relationship Therapy, 30*, 37-59.

Enzlin, P., Mak, R., & Kittel, F., et al. (2004). Sexual functioning in a population-based study of men aged 40-69 years: The good news. *International Journal of Impotence Research, 16*, 512–520.

Erisman, R. (2023). *Cool Facts About The Villages, Florida*. Inside the Bubble: Ultimate Guide to The Villages, FL.

Fernández, J., Marcos, M., & Fernández, C., et al. (2015). The impact of physical exercise on sexual satisfaction. *Psicothema, 27*, 310-315.

Fingerman, L., Pillemer, A., & Silverstein, M., et al. (2012). The Baby Boomers' intergenerational relationships. *Gerontologist, 52*, 199-209.

Flynn, E., Lin, L., & Bruner, W., et al. (2016). Sexual satisfaction and the importance of sexual health to quality of life throughout the life course of U.S. adults. *Journal of Sexual Medicine, 13*, 1642- 1650.

Freak-Poli, R., Kirkman, M., & De Castro Lima, G., et al. (2017). Sexual activity and physical tenderness in older adults: Cross-sectional prevalence and associated characteristics. *Journal of Sexual Medicine, 14*, 918–927.

Gewirtz-Meydan, A., Opuda, E., & Ayalon, L. (2023). Sex and love among older adults in the digital world: A scoping review. *The Gerontologist, 63*, 218–230.

Glass, T. A., de Leon, C. M., & Marottoli, R. A., et al. (1999). Population-based study of social and productive activities as predictors of survival among elderly Americans. *British Medical Journal, 319*, 478.

Grabovac, I., & McDermott, D. T. (2023). Sexuality and sexual activity in older age: An age-old issue? *The Lancet Regional Health. Western Pacific, 39*, 100831.

Gronek, J., Boraczyński, M., & Gronek, P., et al. (2021). Exercise in aging: Be balanced. *Aging and Disabilities, 12*, 1140-1149.

Herrick, L. (2021). Aging and the Sexuality of the Baby Boomers: A Historical and Cultural Examination of "The New Old Age." *In The Palgrave Handbook of Ageing and Physical Activity Promotion*, pp. 353–373. Palgrave Macmillan.

High, C., Fox, J., & McEwan, B. (2024). Technology, relationships, and well-being: An overview of critical research issues and an introduction to the special issue. *Journal of Social and Personal Relationships, 41*, 1055-1072.

Hutto, J., Bell, C., & Farmer, S., et al. (2015). Social media gerontology: Understanding social media usage among older adults. *Web Intelligence and Agent Systems: An International Journal, 13*, 69-87.

Jeannet, M., & Drazanova, L. (2023). Cohort differences in attitudes toward sexual orientation: The formative political climate as a socializing agent. *Frontiers in Political Science, 5*, 1223274. https://doi.org/10.3389/fpos.2023.1223274.

Jenks, R. (1998). Swinging: A review of the literature. *Archives of Sexual Behavior, 27*, 507-521.

Kang, H., & Kim, H. (2022). Ageism and psychological well-being among older adults: A systematic review. *Gerontology and Geriatric Medicine, 8*.

Kotta, S., Ansari, H., & Ali, J. (2013). Exploring scientifically proven herbal aphrodisiacs. *Pharmacology Review, 7*, 1-10.

Kvalem, L., Graham, A., & Hald, M. (2019). The role of body image in sexual satisfaction among partnered older adults: A population-based study in four European countries. *European Journal of Ageing, 17*, 163-173.

Laumann, E., Nicolosi, B., & Glasser, A., et al. (2006). Sexual problems among women and men aged 40–80: Prevalence and correlates identified in the Global Study of Sexual Attitudes and Behaviors. *International Journal of Impotence Research, 18*, 27-39.

Laumann, E., Paik, A., & Rosen, R. (1999). Sexual dysfunction in the United States: Prevalence and predictors. *Journal of the American Medical Association, 28*, 537-544.

Lindau, T., & Gavrilova, N. (2010). Sex, health, and years of sexually active life gained due to good health: Evidence from two U.S. population-based cross-sectional surveys of aging. *British Medical Journal*.

Lindau, T., Schumm, P., & Laumann, E., et al. (2007). A study of sexuality and health among older adults in the United States. *New England Journal of Medicine, 357*, 762-774.

Miguel, I., von Humboldt, S., & Leal, I. (2024). Sexual well-being across the lifespan: Is sexual satisfaction related to adjustment to aging? *Sexual Research and Social Policy*.

Muise, A., Schimmack, U., & Impett, A. (2016). Sexual frequency predicts greater well-being, but more is not always better. *Social Psychological and Personality Science, 7*(4), 295-302.

National Institutes of Health (NIH). (2024). *Sexuality and Intimacy in Older Adults*. National Institute on Aging.

Olshansky, J. (2018). From lifespan to health span. *Journal of the American Medical Association, 320*, 1323–1324.

Ortman, M., Velko, A., & Hogan, H. (2014). *An Aging Nation: The Older Population in the United States*. United States Census Bureau, Economics and Statistics Administration.

Pataky, W., Young, F., & Nair, S. (2021). Hormonal and metabolic changes of aging and the influence of lifestyle modifications. *Mayo Clinic Proceedings, 96*, 788-814.

Penhollow, T. (2007). *Aging and Sexuality: A Study of Active Older Adults*. VDM Verlag Publishing.

Penhollow, T. (2010). *Sexuality, Longevity, and Quality of Life: A Study of America's Largest Active Retirement Community*. VDM Verlag Publishing.

Penhollow, T., Hall, M., & Young, M. (2018). Predictors of sexual satisfaction and self-esteem among active older adults. *International Journal of Health Sciences, 5*, 12-24.

Penhollow, T., Young, M., & Barnes, E. (2022). Perception of person as sexual: View's nursing students have of potential patients. *EC Nursing and Healthcare, 4*, 57-66.

Penhollow, T., Young, M., & Denny, G. (2009). Predictors of quality of life, sexual intercourse, and sexual satisfaction among active older adults. *American Journal of Health Education, 40*, 14-22.

Pew Research Center. (2017). Technology use among seniors. https://www.pewresearch.org/internet/2017/05/17/technologyuse-among-seniors.

Ronghe, V., Pannase, K., & Gomase, K. P., et al. (2023). Understanding hypoactive sexual desire disorder (HSDD) in women: Etiology, diagnosis, and treatment. *Cureus, 15*, e49690. doi: 10.7759/cureus.49690.

Sidoti, O., & Faverio, M. (2023). Dating at 50 and up: Older Americans' experiences with online dating. *Pew Research Center*.

Smith, L., Yang, L., & Veronese, N., et al. (2019). Sexual activity is associated with greater enjoyment of life in older adults. *Sexual Medicine, 7*, 11-18.

Soysal, P., & Avsar, E. (2023). Sexual Activity and Physical Health Benefits in Older Adults. In: Smith, L., Grabovac, I. (eds). *Sexual Behavior and Health in Older Adults. Practical Issues in Geriatrics*.

Stentagg, M., Skär, L., & Berglund, S., et al. (2021). Cross-sectional study of sexual activity and satisfaction among older adults≥60 years of age. *Sexual Medicine, 9*, 100316.

Stowell, M., Hall, A., & Warwick, S. (2023). Promoting sexual health in older adults: Findings from two rapid reviews. *Maturitas, 177*.

United States Census Bureau. (2024). *The Population 65 Years and Older: 2021.*

Uzdavines, A., Helmer, A., & Spelman, F. (2022). Sexual health assessment is vital to whole health models of care. *Journal of Medical Internet Research, 3*:e36266.

Waite, J., Duvoisin, R., & Kotwal, A. (2021). Social Health in the National Social Life, Health, and Aging Project. *The Journals of Gerontology: Series B, 76,* S251-S265.

Wilkowska, W., Brauner, P., & Ziee, M. (2018). Rethinking technology development for older adults: A responsible research and innovation duty. *Aging, Technology and Health,* 1-30.

Woloski-Wruble, C., Oliel, Y., & Leefsma, M. (2010). Sexual activities, sexual and life satisfaction, and successful aging in women. *Journal of Sexual Medicine, 7,* 2401–2410.

Zhang, F., Yang, Z., & Li, X., et al. (2023). Factors influencing the quality of sexual life in the older adults: A scoping review. *International Journal of Nursing and Science, 10,* 167-173.

Resources

Education and Support

1. American Sexual Health Association (ASHA)

- **Website:** https://www.ashasexualhealth.org
- **Services:** ASHA offers resources on sexual health throughout life, covering topics like aging, STIs, and sexual function. They provide educational materials, support hotlines, and help locate healthcare providers.

2. The North American Menopause Society (NAMS)

- **Website:** https://www.menopause.org
- **Services:** NAMS focuses on menopause and health for midlife women, including sexual health. Their resources include information on hormone therapy, sexual function, and overall wellness during aging.

3. SAGE (Services & Advocacy for GLBT Elders)

- **Website:** https://www.sageusa.org
- **Services:** SAGE supports and advocates for LGBTQ+ older adults. Their resources address aging, including sexual health, mental health, and social support.

4. AARP (American Association of Retired Persons)

- **Website:** https://www.aarp.org
- **Services:** AARP offers a wide range of articles, resources, and guides, including sexual health specifically for older adults. AARP also has forums for discussions and support on various health-related topics.

5. International Society for Sexual Medicine (ISSM)

- **Website:** https://www.issm.info
- **Services:** ISSM offers research, education, and resources on sexual health, including age-related issues. ISSM provides information for both medical professionals and patients on sexual dysfunction and treatment options.

6. Mayo Clinic

- **Website:** https://www.mayoclinic.org
- **Services:** Mayo Clinic provides comprehensive health information, including topics on sexual health and aging. They offer articles and expert advice on maintaining sexual health, managing chronic conditions, and understanding changes in sexual function.

7. Planned Parenthood

- **Website:** https://www.plannedparenthood.org
- **Services:** Planned Parenthood offers educational resources and healthcare services related to sexual health for all ages, including older adults. They provide information on sexual health, safe sex practices, and access to healthcare providers.

8. Healthy Aging

- **Website:** https://healthyaging.net
- **Services:** Healthy Aging promotes positive aging with resources on sexual health, mental well-being, and overall wellness for older adults. They provide articles, webinars, and expert advice covering various aspects of aging.

9. American Geriatrics Society (AGS)

- **Website:** https://www.americangeriatrics.org

- **Services:** AGS offers resources and research on health issues affecting older adults, including sexual health. They provide clinical guidelines, patient information, and educational materials for healthcare providers and older adults.

10. Centers of Disease Control and Prevention (CDC)

- **Website:** https://www.cdc.gov
- **Services:** The CDC provides comprehensive information on sexual health, including disease prevention, STIs, contraception, and general public health guidelines. It also offers educational resources, statistics, and recommendations for maintaining sexual wellness and preventing the spread of infections.

Sex Therapy and Counseling

1. American Association of Sexuality Educators, Counselors, and Therapists (ASSECT)

- **Website:** https://www.aasect.org
- **Services:** AASECT provides a directory of certified sex therapists, counselors, and educators to help individuals and couples improve their sexual health and relationships. The organization also offers professional training and certification for individuals in the fields of sexuality education, therapy, and counseling.

Sex Toys

1. Senior Planet

- **Website:** https://seniorplanet.org
- **Overview:** Senior Planet, an initiative by Older Adults Technology Services (OATS), offers a variety of articles on technology and lifestyle topics for older adults. They include open discussions on sexual wellness and the use of sex toys.

2. Smitten Kitten

- **Website:** https://www.smittenkittenonline.com
- **Overview:** Smitten Kitten is an educational and shopping website focused on sex toys for older adults. It features high-quality products and provides educational resources that emphasize the benefits of sex toys, with a focus on comfort, ease of use, and safety.

3. Scarleteen

- **Website:** https://www.scarleteen.com
- **Overview:** Scarleteen, while primarily targeting younger audiences, offers inclusive sexual health education that includes discussions about sex toys. The site provides valuable information relevant to people of all ages, including older adults.

4. OMGYes

- **Website:** https://start.omgyes.com
- **Overview:** OMGYes is dedicated to women's sexual pleasure, offering research-backed insights that can be particularly beneficial for older women interested in exploring sex toys to enhance their sexual experiences.

5. Lovehoney

- **Website:** https://www.lovehoney.com
- **Overview:** Lovehoney is a well-known online retailer offering a broad selection of sex toys. The site provides detailed product descriptions and customer reviews, helping older adults find items that suit their needs, including options for those with mobility issues or sensitivity concerns.

6. Adam & Eve

- **Website:** https://www.adameve.com

- **Overview:** Adam & Eve is one of the largest online retailers for adult products, offering a wide selection of sex toys and related items. The site provides guides to help customers select products that are comfortable and effective across different age groups.

7. Good Vibrations

- **Website:** https://www.goodvibes.com
- **Overview:** Good Vibrations is known for its educational approach to sexual wellness, offering a variety of sex toys with an emphasis on inclusivity. It serves as a valuable resource for older adults seeking products that are safe and easy to use.

8. Babeland

- **Website:** https://www.babeland.com
- **Overview:** Babeland offers a range of sex toys and accessories, focusing on education and inclusivity. The site provides information on selecting toys particularly suitable for older adults, including those experiencing changes in sexual function due to aging.

Senior Sites

1. Sixty and Me

- **Website:** https://www.sixtyandme.com
- **Overview:** Sixty and Me is an online magazine aimed at women over 60, offering articles, videos, and resources on topics like health, wellness, relationships, and retirement. It also provides practical tips on aging gracefully, staying active, and maintaining a positive outlook on life.

2. Suddenly Senior

- **Website:** https://www.suddenlysenior.com
- **Overview:** Suddenly Senior is a humorous and insightful website dedicated to seniors. It offers a mix of jokes, nostalgia, and practical

advice on aging, health, and retirement. The site provides articles on relationships, healthcare, money-saving tips, and senior advocacy, blending humor and useful information to entertain and inform older adults.

3. Senior Journal

- **Website:** http://www.seniorjournal.com
- **Overview:** Senior Journal is an online news source focused on providing relevant and up-to-date information for seniors. It covers a wide range of topics including health, retirement, Medicare, Social Security, and aging-related legislative changes. The site offers articles on scientific advancements, caregiving, senior rights, and wellness tips.

Acknowledgments

I extend my deepest gratitude to the following individuals and groups whose contributions have been invaluable to completing this book project.

First and foremost, I am profoundly grateful to my parents for their unwavering support, encouragement, and love. Your belief in my abilities has been a constant source of motivation and strength. Thank you for always being there for me and providing a solid foundation during my challenges and successes. Your guidance, wisdom, and faith have been the cornerstone of everything I've achieved.

I would also like to extend my deepest thanks to Dr. Young, my mentor, who inspired and encouraged me to pursue the field of sexual health science. Your insightful guidance and unwavering support have shaped my academic journey and personal growth. The knowledge and wisdom you shared, along with your dedication to my development, have been instrumental in helping me reach this milestone.

Lastly, I offer my sincere appreciation to the residents of The Villages for their enthusiastic participation in my research over the years. Your willingness to share your personal stories, behaviors, and experiences has been invaluable to my work and has made a meaningful impact on the broader understanding of sexual health and wellness. Through your openness and trust, this book has become a powerful reflection of your lived realities and insights.

I express my heartfelt gratitude to all of you—I am forever thankful.

About The Author

Tina M. Penhollow, Ph.D., MCHES is a non-fiction author and health behavior scientist with expertise in sexual health, aging, exercise, and wellness. With over two decades of research on how aging impacts intimacy and overall quality of life, she is dedicated to helping older adults thrive by offering knowledge, strategies, and resources for aging with vitality, confidence, and fulfillment.

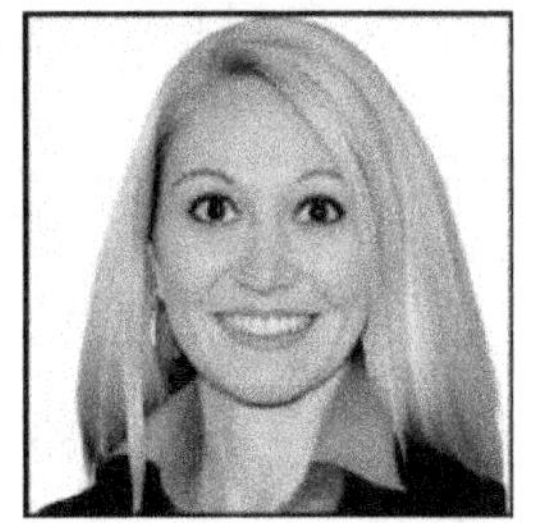

As one of the early pioneers to achieve the distinction of Master Certified Health Education Specialist (MCHES), her work has been widely published in academic journals and prominent online publications. Her insights have been featured in outlets such as *The London Times*, *The Los Angeles Times*, *Women's Health*, *Cosmopolitan*, *Glamour*, and *Shape*.

Dr. Penhollow is a health science professor at Florida Atlantic University in Boca Raton, where she is dedicated to educating and inspiring the future generation of health professionals. Outside the classroom, she loves unwinding on the golf course and spending quality time with her family and beloved dog, Maverick.

Discover more about her work and insights at drtinapenhollow.com

9 798999 147399 6